Vagus Nerve Exercises to Rewire Your Brain

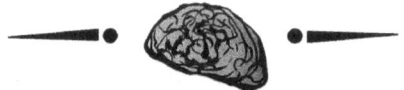

Discover Science-Backed Methods to Activate or Reset
Your Vagus Nerve. Transform Your Life with Polyvagal Exercises
to Reduce Anxiety and Heal from Trauma

Tom Baily

Copyright © 2024 by Tom Baily
All rights reserved.

It is illegal to reproduce, duplicate, or transmit any part of this document in any form, electronic or printed. Recording or storing this document is prohibited without written permission from the publisher, except for brief quotations in a book review.

No responsibility will be held against the publisher or author for any damages or losses due to the information in this book. You are responsible for your own actions and results.

Legal Notice:

This book is copyright protected and for personal use only. You cannot amend, distribute, sell, use, quote, or paraphrase any part of this book without consent from the author or publisher.

Disclaimer Notice:

The information in this document is for educational and entertainment purposes only. All efforts have been made to ensure accurate and complete information. No warranties are implied. The author is not giving legal, financial, medical, or professional advice. Content has been derived from various sources. Consult a licensed professional before attempting any techniques in this book.

By reading this document, you agree that the author is not responsible for any losses due to the use of the information, including errors, omissions, or inaccuracies.

ISBN: 9798328445375

Contents

Introduction	1
1. Anatomy and Functions of the Vagus Nerve	6
2. An Introduction to Polyvagal Theory	21
3. The Vagus Nerve's Role in Anxiety, Trauma, and Stress	34
4. Breathing Exercises to Stimulate the Vagus Nerve	41
5. Mindfulness and Meditation Practices for Vagal Tone	56
6. Yoga Poses and Sequences to Tone the Vagus Nerve	75
7. Sound Therapy and Chanting for Vagus Nerve Stimulation	100
8. Acupressure and Massage Techniques for the Vagus Nerve	126
9. Cold Exposure and Hydrotherapy for Vagus Nerve Activation	134
10. Laughter, Singing, and Gargling for Vagus Nerve Stimulation	142
11. Nutrition and Diet for Optimal Vagus Nerve Function	151
12. Exercise and Physical Activity for Vagus Nerve Stimulation	157
13. Sleep and Circadian Rhythm for Vagus Nerve Health	169

14. Stress Management and Relaxation Techniques for Vagal Tone   181

15. Creating a Daily Vagus Nerve Exercise Routine   189

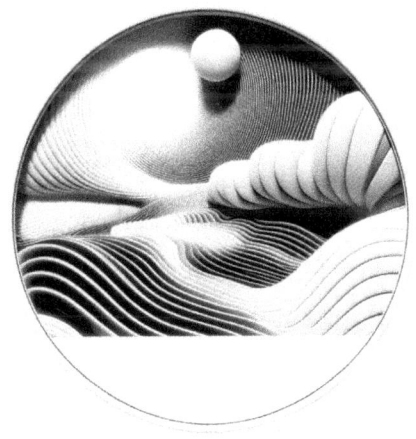

Introduction

Welcome to this incredible journey of discovery into the transformational power of the vagus nerve. If you are just like so many others who have been suffering or struggling with anxiety, chronic stress, or trauma, then with this book, you will have all that you need to go through these adversities and balance vigor back in your life. My name is Tom Baly, and from personal experience with the power of the Vagus nerve, I am so excited to share knowledge and practices that I know have transformed my life and many others.

Imagine activating your natural "parasympathetic brake system" on-demand, returning you to that state of calm and balance quickly when stress hits. Imagine living resiliently—connected and filled with lasting joy—while dwelling on the messiness that life can deliver. I can make those words come true by releasing and toning the vagus nerve, our most potent ally in attaining complete health. It is only because I have spent years digging deep and have doggedly practiced and taught with great passion that I have brought to my understanding the tremendous potency of this nerve in revolutionizing the life experience of human beings.

In this revolutionary book, "Vagus Nerve Exercises to Rewire Your Brain", I'll be taking you by your hand, step by step, through this fascinating world of this incredible bundle of nerve fibers, revealing how you can harness its full potential to transform your life from the inside out. If you are dealing with gut-wrenching anxiety, burnout that leaves you bone-tired, or the lingering dopo effetto of trauma, this book gives you pragmatic techniques and exercises that you can use to heal yourself from the inside out to start leading a life full of joy from living all over again.

We'll soon dive into the transformative practices, but before that, I consider it crucial to understand how fundamentally important this nerve is to your overall well-being. This excellent nerve happens to be the longest in the autonomic nervous system, and it acts as a vital bridge between the brain and the body, playing extensively into digestion, heart rate, immune response, and emotional processing. Telling the stories of personal transformation, ancient wisdom, and cutting-edge scientific research shows how the vagus nerve emotionally mediates between the mind and the body to modulate and promote physical health.

A sense of quietness, centeredness in the core, and robustness develops to face life's challenges when the vagus is healthy and in harmony. It gives us the capacity to navigate through life's challenges with grace, flexibility, and wisdom. When chronic stress or unresolved traumas are part of this history, our nervous system can become taken hostage in the state of hypervigilance or shut down emotionally, hijacking this flexibility to be relaxed, open to others, and vibrantly alive.

This is where the groundbreaking polyvagal theory, masterfully developed by luminary Dr. Stephen Porges, comes alive as a lens through which one can understand the intricate dance between the vagus nerve and our autonomic nervous system. This pioneering theory lays bare how, interacting with the sympathetic and parasympathetic branches, the vagus nerve shapes our emotional, cognitive, and physiological experiences from moment to moment. It provides a potent map between the various states of our nervous system, which range from calm connection to sympathetic activation in a "fight or flight" response and into the states of freeze and dissociation. It teaches us how to construct a state of safety and social engagement. We will learn how to purposefully activate the vagus nerve in a targeted way so we can access our built-in parasympathetic brake. So we can soothe an over-cranked nervous system and reclaim a deep sense of inner safety, authentic connection, and well-being.

But this book is not just a theoretical exercise. It is an invitation to actualization and transformation. We will use a variety of practical exercises and proven techniques, as explained in the first section, ranging from mindful breathing with yoga, meditation, and cold exposure to singing and massage. You will learn to work with your nervous system in new, empowering ways. Whether you are an inquisitive newcomer or someone with years of experience in the field, you tend to find natural tools that can easily slip into your daily life. I'll gently lead you through each practice with clear and accessible instructions—adapting it for different abilities and needs—and how to work through common problems.

Here is a summary of the journey of transformation that awaits you:

In Part I, "Understanding the Vagus Nerve and Polyvagal Theory," we will take a deep dive into the anatomy and functioning of the vagus nerve as a basic understanding of this all-important system. Learn about the vagus nerve's role in mood regulations, digestion, heart rate, the immune system, and many other things. We will also further expand upon the groundbreaking Polyvagal Theory, which will be the guiding map for our explorations of the states of our nervous systems in our journey toward safety and connection. We'll learn what the vagus nerve has to do with experiencing anxiety, trauma, and stress and how the Polyvagal Theory guides that paradigm regarding healing and growth.

Part II, "Vagus Nerve Exercises and Techniques", is the practical toolbox of exercises to stimulate and tone the vagus nerve: movement, breath, meditation, sound, and more. Beginning with pranayama and diaphragmatic breathing exercises, powerful practices of breath include a relaxing as well as energizing sequence of yoga and mindfulness exercises building up momentary awareness. You can physically feel the transformation that arises from these practices. We will also look at how to bring in massage techniques, cold exposure, chanting, gargling, and even laughter in ways that powerfully stimulate the vagus nerve.

Lifestyle Practices for Vagal Tone: Part III: Long-Term Lifestyle Practices That Are Pro-Vagal Nerve Health and Resilience. We will be learning how our food, physical activity, rest, sleep, social relationships, and stress management all play a core, supporting role in the proper vagal tone for us in general with our health and well-being. I will show you how to create a personal road map for integrating these foundational practices into your daily routine, taking into account your unique preferences and circumstances.

Finally, in Part IV, "Incorporating Vagus Nerve Exercises into Daily Life," you will learn how to make vagus nerve stimulation practices a natural part of your daily existence and life. You will design a training program tailored to you, get and stay motivated, avoid or overcome common obstacles, and track your progress over time. We will also explore the application of vagus-stimulating exercises across life contexts, emotions, and phases of development—from distressing states of anxiety and panic to supporting experiences of happiness and other positive emotions.

Read on if you are prepared to take your healing, self-discovery, and transformational journey. Wisdom from the polyvagal theory to guide us and the power of exercises for the vagus nerve to move us—we have all we need to unlock our full potential for health, resilience, and vitality. From here, your healing and growth story goes on; this is how the endless possibilities we hold together can be changed.

With gratitude, compassion, and an unwavering belief that you are healed

Tom Baily

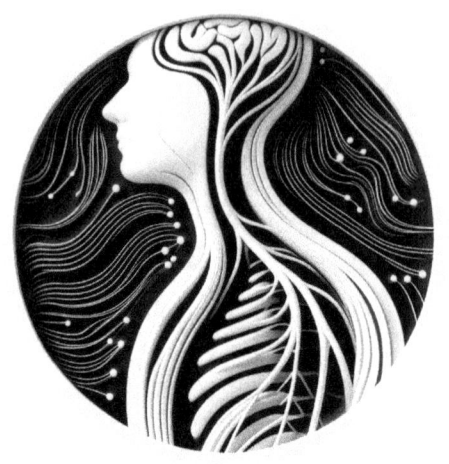

Chapter 1
Anatomy and Functions of the Vagus Nerve

Consider your body as a vast, symphonic orchestra with many different organs playing their particular song, and at the center, the conductor—a vagal conductor. This excellent nerve fiber transmission goes from the brain to the viscera and orchestrates all those life processes that help us feel good.

In this chapter, we will set the stage by looking at the anatomy and function of the vagus nerve, and it will become apparent that the pitcher said component of the ANS is intimately connected about physical, emotional, and social health. Find that the vagus nerve truly bridges the autonomic nervous system, the heart, the digestive system, and the immune system in modulating the stress response and the growth of resilience.

In the stories of transformation and practical examples, we will show the power of the vagus nerve in healing and balance in such conditions as anxiety and depression to digestive and autoimmune diseases. We will provide concrete strategies for the assessment and strengthening of vagal function: deep breathing to self-regulation techniques.

Now, on this journey of discovery, I want you to open your mind and come to this material with great curiosity. If you are looking to optimize your well-being, overcome chronic health challenges, or simply deepen your understanding of the body's innate wisdom, the insights, and practices in this book can potentially transform your life.

Remember, restorations and the re-building of resilience are often non-linear processes. It is made up of a few significant breakthroughs, with a few setbacks as well. Yet, like any skill, over time, with practice, self-compassion, and belief in the ability to entrust the body to make its way back to balance and even healing through the process of finding it, you will be able to build a robust and responsive vagus—an inner conductor watching over you toward harmony and health.

So take a deep breath, tune in with the wisdom of your body, and let's begin this journey into the extraordinary world of the vagus nerve.

1.1 The Vagus Nerve: A Key Component of the Autonomic Nervous System

It plays a central role in the autonomic nervous system—the vagus nerve is the longest and most complex of the cranial nerves. The ANS controls all the involuntary functions in your body, such as heart rate, digestion, and respiration. The two divisions are the sympathetic nervous system (SNS), which is the "fight or flight" system, and the parasympathetic nervous system (PNS). The vagus nerve makes up the central part of the PNS and is considered to act as a brake in counterbalance to the accelerating effect of the SNS.

During stress, the SNS elicits a "fight-or-flight" reaction: it raises heart rate and blood pressure and redirects blood flow to the muscles. Once the stressor leaves, the vagus nerve lowers heart rate and blood pressure, returning the body to a calm, relaxed state. This "rest-and-digest" response is essential for maintaining homeostasis and keeping the destructive effects of chronic stress at bay.

The influence of the vagal nerve is much more than just the regulator of the stress response—it reaches the heart, the lungs, the stomach, the intestines, and even the immune system. The Vagus nerve regulates their activity to keep the body's internal balance intact. Therefore, the vagus nerve, via its extensive connections, shares high importance to physical and emotional well-being.

Consider, for example, Emily, a young woman who suffered from chronic anxiety and panic attacks. The assessment would quickly reveal her vagal tone to be extremely low, probably due to several very early life stressors combined with her frenzied, high-pressure lifestyle. Through concerted practitioner guidance, deep breathing, meditation, and self-regulating techniques within a structured vagal nerve exercise routine, Emily was pulled into much amelioration of her symptoms. At that moment, she said, she felt more centered, stronger, and able to quickly deal with whatever life presented.

However, the vagus nerve does not use its powers for the sake of promoting healing and resilience in the arena of mental health alone. Studies indicate that vagal tone stands out among the best predictors of cardiovascular health and that higher vagal activity results in a lessened risk of heart disease, stroke, and other cardiovascular events. A vital and responsive vagus is cultivated through proper exercises and lifestyle changes that garner health and vitality in the heart.

At each step into the world of the vagus nerve, it becomes pretty clear that this incredible nerve is one of the master regulators of our health. We can come to understand some of its functioning and learn how to support its good condition to gain access to another vital source of healing and resilience.

1.2 The Parasympathetic and Sympathetic Nervous Systems: A Delicate Dance

Appreciation of the significance of the vagus nerve is an understanding of the functional cooperation of the parasympathetic and sympathetic nervous systems. The harmonious work of these two divisions of the autonomic nervous system helps in the maintenance of the balance of life and adaptiveness to the constantly changing demands of the inner and outer world.

The SNS involves the body's "accelerator," mediating the "fight-or-flight" response. When a challenge or physical threat is detected, the body quickly increases the heart rate and blood pressure and shunts blood to the working muscles. These states prepare our bodies in arousal, which become essential for survival by responding appropriately and effectively to danger.

Conversely, the PNS, driven by the vagus nerve, works as a "brake" for the body. The vagus nerve, after the passing of the threat, slows down the heart rate and blood pressure in the body and encourages relaxation and restoration. This "rest-and-digest" response is essential in the resource recovery and homeostasis of the body to effect repair, healing, and recharge.

It is the balance between the SNS and PNS that maintains health and life in the body. Disruption in the balance between these two systems—when one overpowers the other—creates the breeding ground for severe complications. However, chronic stress that represents continuous SNS activation and PNS underactivity is likely to be implicated in a wide range of health problems, including anxiety, depression, digestive issues, and low immune defense.

This is where the power of targeted vagus nerve exercises comes into play. Anything that tends to strengthen vagal tones through deep diaphragmatic breathing, meditation, and self-regulation techniques reinstates the balance between the SNS and PNS. Improvements to our vagal tone enhance resistance to the stress response, emotional regulation, and general health and vitality.

Take the case of John, an executive under great tension who was on the verge of burnout. Years of exposure to chronic stress had sapped his general health, and symptoms of high blood pressure, insomnia, and constant anxiety plagued his life. But when he went through a holistic program of vagal nerve stimulation that includes regular breathing exercises, cold water therapy, and mindfulness practices, John started experiencing a state of being radically different in terms of his well-being. His blood pressure came back to normalcy, he slept well, and he had an increase in confidence to face the experiments at the workplace.

The dance between the SNS and the PNS orchestrated by the vagus nerve is a beautiful example of the body's innate wisdom and capacity for self-regulation. Cultivating a good, strong, and responsive vagus nerve allows for the refinement of the balance that supports health, resiliency, and vitality in all aspects of our lives.

1.3 The Vagus Nerve's Role in Emotional Regulation

One of the most exciting things is that the vagus nerve hugely impacts our emotional lives. Recently, emerging research has found the vagus nerve to be a critical factor in controlling emotion, shaping our stress responses, and promoting resilience.

It is the central bi-directional relay between the body and the limbic area of the brain, represented by the amygdala and prefrontal cortex, with an essential role in executive function. Therefore, it sends information from the body to the brain about the internal environment, a change which eventually leads to an alteration in the emotional state and a change in the response of an organism to stress. In turn, the brain can use the vagus nerve to modulate the body's physiological state, inducing a state of calm and relaxation in times of distress.

It is this intimate connection of the vagus nerve to emotional regulation that the renowned Dr. Stephen Porges developed in his polyvagal theory. The theory puts forth that the health and tone of our vagus nerve determines, to a more significant extent, positive social interactions and opportunities regarding emotional regulation. High vagal tone is frequently associated with high emotional resilience, good stress management, and satisfying relationships.

This little organ, the vagus nerve, forms the powerhouse of emotional regulation—not so evident until one loses the use of the vagal brake, a force dramatically shown by the case of Sophie, a young woman with severe social anxiety that afflicted her existence. For many years, Sophie remained paralyzed by that vicious cycle of self-criticism and avoided situations where she might become connected with others. She started to notice a difference in her emotional landscape after following a targeted program of vagal exercises that included deep breathing, chanting, and self-compassion practices. She felt more grounded, self-assured, and able to navigate social interactions with much ease and confidence.

A robust and responsive vagus nerve supports emotional resilience, which in turn helps mental well-being. The higher vagal tone has reduced depression and anxiety disorders in study after study. With training in techniques that increase vagal tone—like meditation, yoga, and expressive writing—we may create states of emotional equilibrium, psychological flexibility, and a sense of inner peace.

The parasympathetic nervous system - the vagus nerve, functioning in emotion regulation - embraces social connection and empathy. Another aspect that makes the vagus nerve so important concerns the "neural underpinning of the social engagement system," a term used by Dr. Porges to describe the neural circuitry through which we interact with others and our emotional lives are co-regulated. When we interact with others in a positive social manner, such as making eye contact, listening to what they say, or sharing a warm embrace, we stimulate the system, converting such feelings into those of safety, trust, and belonging.

By nurturing our vagus nerve and building a robust social engagement system, we can then further upregulate our capacity to be empathic, compassionate, and genuinely connected with others. This will benefit not only the personal relations of the people involved but also the creation of a more empathetic and strong society overall.

The more we study the vagus in the context of emotional regulation, the more we realize that this astonishing nerve forms the key to unlocking our potential for a healthy life and flourishing relationships. By incorporating practices that support vagal health and being more aware of our emotional landscape, we move through life's challenges with more resilience, grace, and heart.

1.4 The Role of the Vagus Nerve in Digestion and Gut Health

The vagus nerve, often called the "wear-and-ging nerve," is responsible for more than just regulating emotions and how you respond to stress. This master regulator coordinates the complex functions of the digestive system, including the absorption of nutrients, gut motility, and inflammation.

The digestive system contains a surprising amount of neurons, often referred to as the "second brain" or enteric nervous system. The conduit of information flow is by the vagus nerve between such plexuses and the central nervous system, which serves for information integration with constant connection and guarantees the regulation of internal organs. Such bidirectional communication is essential for proper functioning in everyday life.

Among the most critical roles of the vagus nerve in digestion is controlling the motility of the gastrointestinal system. The vagus nerve stimulates the smooth muscles of the digestive tract, raising peristalsis—the movements pushing food through the esophagus, stomach, and intestines. These peristaltic movements are appropriately coordinated and effective in the best vagal tone in consideration of proper digestion and absorption of nutrients.

However, the insufficiency of vagal function can lead to digestive disorders. Poor vagal tone has been implicated in a wide variety of pathologies within the GI tract, from IBS to IBD and gastroparesis. In this case, symptoms include bloating, abdominal pain, constipation, and diarrhea.

The tale of Michael, who suffered from chronic digestive disorders, is a recuperative story with sufficient vigor of supportive vagal nerve function. Michael had been having frequent complaints of abdominal pain, bloating, and irregular bowel habits that hampered the quality of his life for years. The evaluation showed that the vagal tone was poor in Michael, probably due to chronic stress and a history of antibiotic use.

By re-activating his vagus with a program of targeted vagus exercises, including deep belly breathing, humming, and gargling, Michael experienced a dramatic change in his digestive symptoms. He now had less bloating, more regular bowel movements, and felt much more comfortable and at ease in his gut. Of course, all this not only physically improved his well-being but made a considerable change upward in his emotional tone and general quality of life.

More recently, the influence of the vagus nerve on the state of the gut extends far beyond simple motility control. One of the more exceptional roles of this nerve is to have a vital role in the modulation of inflammation and immune function within the gut. The vagus nerve is part of an "inflammatory reflex" that may help control the inflammatory reaction of the whole body.

The vagus nerve detected the inflammatory signals within the gut and relayed the information to the brain to mediate an anti-inflammatory response. It is mediated by the release of acetylcholine, a neurotransmitter, acting on the acetylcholine receptor in immune cells by suppressing the synthesis of pro-inflammatory cytokines. Consequently, the vagus nerve keeps a handle on the inflammation, thus maintaining an appropriate balance in the gut, circumvents chronic inflammatory pathologies.

By supporting the vagal tone with specific exercises and lifestyle modifications, gut health improvement can be gained and overall well-being enhanced. Direct improvements to vagal function and gut-brain axis health have been identified with mind-body approaches to eating—such as yoga and tai chi. Improvement in digestion and the enhancement of gastrointestinal resilience are continued with a diet high in gut-supportive nutrients and probiotics.

As we continue to unlock the complex relationship between the vagus nerve and gut health, it becomes more apparent that it is the nurturing of this vital connection that may well hold the secret to good digestion and overall well-being. Engaging with these practices that support vagal tone and a healthy gut-brain axis creates a digestive system more nutritious, more balanced, and more resilient, forming the core foundation of a lifetime of health and vitality.

1.5 The Role of the Vagus Nerve on the Heart and Respiratory System

In the great symphony of the human body, the vagus nerve emerges as a master conductor orchestrating the intricate functions of two of our most vital systems: the cardiovascular and respiratory systems. Through its far-reaching fibers, the vagus nerve is placed in a central role in regulating heart rate, blood pressure, and breathing patterns with efforts at harmonious and adaptive responsiveness to the ever-changing demands in the environment.

Perhaps the most interesting connection of the vagus is with the heart. The incredible vagus nerve supplies the sinoatrial node—the natural pacemaker of the heart—enabling the constant modulation of the rate of heartbeat to fluctuations in inner and environmental demand. Activation of the vagus nerve will send signals to the heart to slow down, inducing relaxation and calm. This 'vagal brake' is a significant key to the maintenance of cardiovascular health and prevention of deleterious effects due to chronic stress and sympathetic overactivation.

These findings have kind of of underlined the importance of vagal tone in the health of the cardiovascular system because they gave way to the concept of heart rate variability (HRV). HRV is the variation in time between one heartbeat and the next beat, reflecting the capacity of the organism for adaptation to changes in stressor demands or environmental conditions. High HRV, signifying high variability between beats, has been taken as a measurement of good vagal tone and good cardiovascular flexibility. In contrast, low HRV implies poor vagal function and low adaptability in the individual, which goes further to increases the risks of several cardiovascular diseases, anxiety, and depression.

Strength and improvement in vagus nerve responsiveness through specialized exercises and lifestyle interventions are vital to cardiovascular health. Deep breathing, meditation, and yoga all elevate HRV and vagal tone, which cultivates resiliency and adaptability in the cardiovascular system. Making these practices part of our daily lives can be crucial in promoting good cardiovascular health, possibly reducing the possibility of becoming ill from cardiovascular disease and, therefore, promoting general well-being.

The influence of the vagus nerve on the breathing system is equally impressive. This jaw-dropping nerve supplies the muscles of the throat, larynx, and bronchi, which help the process of breathing and the exchange of oxygen and carbon dioxide. When one inhales, the vagus nerve signals the diaphragm and intercostal muscles to enable the lungs to expand and aid in the intake of oxygen-rich air. The vagus nerve controls this muscle action during exhalation so that the air loaded with carbon dioxide can be pushed out.

Beyond just its mechanical role in respiration, the vagus nerve is also a key component in integrating our breath with our heartbeat—an interaction sometimes referred to as "cardiorespiratory coupling." The time of active vagal activity is reduced somewhat during an inhaled breath, thereby creating a distinct increase in heart rate. During expiration, a boost in vagal activity is given, thus causing a distinct slowing of the heart. Rhythmic entrainment of breath and heartbeat ensures efficiency in gas exchange and blood flow optimization, so every cell is well nourished and oxygenated to the optimal amount.

The yogic art of breath control, or Pranayama, is another beautiful practice that illustrates the power of the vagus nerve in respiratory health. It takes deep, slow, and rhythmic patterns in inspiration and expiration that stimulate the vagus nerve to maintain relaxation, clarity, and poise. Clinical and experimental studies have shown that individuals who regularly practice pranayama have a marked improvement in their respiratory functions, cardiovascular health, and overall well-being.

1.6 The Vagus Nerve and Immune Function

The vagus emerges in the health and protection tapestry of our body and mind as a potent ally in the quest for optimal immune function and resilience. This extraordinary, far-reaching nerve of profound effects plays a central role in modulating immune responses and the inflammatory balance.

This provides a critical link of communication between the brain and the immune system, hence enabling an unceasing back-and-forth flow of information between these two major adaptive systems. With this sophisticated pathway of signaling, the vagus nerve detects the presence of pathogens, inflammatory cytokines, and other kinds of danger signals within the internal milieu of the body. It conveys this critical information to the brain, which would serve in waking up appropriate immune and behavioral responses through raising alarms that fit the occasion.

On the other hand, the vagus nerve can be availed to send commands from the brain to the immune system, thus effectively affecting the peripheral factors' influence, such as stress, emotions, or thoughts. This top-down control allows the central regulation of immune response to be fine-tuned such that the changes are appropriate to the developing needs of the body.

Of particular interest is the vagus nerve's anti-inflammatory role, at least in part through an "inflammatory reflex." This powerful feedback loop, hence orchestrated by the vagus nerve, helps to calibrate inflammation, avoiding overactive immune reactions that can harm healthy tissues.

Some of the inflammatory molecules that the vagus nerve will detect circulating levels of are TNF-alpha and interleukin-6—and it sends a signal to the brain to turn the off switch of the inflammatory arm of the parasympathetic nervous system. In turn, it activates the release of acetylcholine, a neurotransmitter that binds to receptors on immune cells, especially the macrophage—the clean-up crew of the immune system.

This mechanism calms an inflammatory response by reducing the release of proinflammatory cytokines through the action of acetylcholine on phagocytes' receptors. This "brake" system driven by the vagus ultimately serves the function of minimizing collateral damage to the host and facilitating inflammation resolution post-threat clearance.

Implications of the inflammatory reflex go well beyond the field of immunity or even biology in general. Otherwise defined as an overzealous and persistent immune response, chronic inflammation lies at the root of conditions as diverse as diabetes, heart disease, and many disabling disorders, including autoimmune diseases and neurodegenerative diseases. Unraveling and harnessing the anti-inflammatory power of the vagus nerve might offer new and promising approaches for preventing and curing such disorders.

Further interventions in lifestyle to support an increased vagal tone would have a powerful effect on regulating immunity and the balance of inflammation. Deep diaphragmatic breathing, meditation, and self-regulation techniques are vaunted for their capacity to bring about immune balance and resilience by enhancing vagal function. Such practices further improve the vagus, providing a state of security with constant vigilance. This environment is functional for the immune system and general well-being.

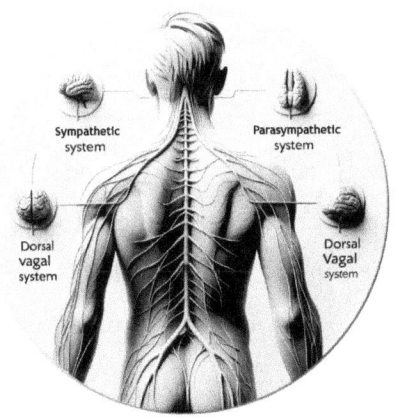

Chapter 2
An Introduction to Polyvagal Theory

Few structures are more central to our well-being and vitality in the vast landscape of our human experience than the autonomic nervous system, spreading this remarkable nerve tissue and control center in nearly every organ and tissue of the body. Orchestrating functions that maintain life itself, the autonomic nervous system fills this very foundational role, although it is often misunderstood and oversimplified.

Thanks to the work of Dr. Stephen Porges and his Polyvagal Theory: we now have a much deeper understanding of the ANS as a far more nuanced and hierarchically organized system than we ever expected. This pioneering conceptual framework revolutionized the experience of the relations of the autonomic nervous system with human emotions and social behavior.

In this chapter, we will delve into the roots of Polyvagal Theory as we reveal the three hierarchically organized subsystems of the ANS and how it guides our experience from one moment to the next. We will dissect the operations of the ventral vagal complex and the social-engagement system, as well as the operations of the sympathetic nervous system and the mobilization response and how the dorsal vagal complex is linked to the immobilization responses. And then, we can talk about neuroception and how we create a sense of safety and find danger in the world.

As we embark on this discovery journey, I urge you to do so with curiosity and an open heart. Each insight, even if small relative to the large picture, that Polyvagal Theory provides can be transformational in creating new perspectives on oneself and others, thus offering a robust frame for one to consider resilience, connection, and well-being in life.

2.1 The Origins of Polyvagal Theory

Polyvagal Theory, developed by renowned researcher Dr. Stephen Porges, signifies a paradigm shift in our appreciation of the autonomic nervous system and its interface with human behavior and experience. This groundbreaking framework emerged from decades of rigorous research in neuroscience, psychophysiology, and evolutionary biology.

Fundamental to Polyvagal Theory is the conception that the autonomic nervous system is organized into three distinct subsystems, each with unique functions and evolutionary origins. The subsystems are hierarchically organized as the ventral vagal complex related to social engagement, the sympathetic nervous system related to mobilization, and the dorsal vagal complex related to immobilization.

Porges identified the critical involvement of the vagus nerve, the tenth cranial nerve, in mediating these autonomic states and behavioral responses. He identified that the vagus nerve is not one nerve, but it is made up of two separate pathways: the ventral vagal path, derived from the nucleus ambiguus, and the dorsal vagal pathway, derived from the dorsal motor nucleus.

This anatomical distinction then forms the basis for a polyvagal hierarchy, with the ventral vagal complex representing the most evolved and advanced system for regulating physiological states and social behavior. When the ventral vagal complex is optimally working and active, we experience feelings of safety, connection, and engagement with others.

However, when danger or harm is imminent or under adversity, the autonomic nervous system can become dominated by the sympathetic nervous system, mobilizing the body through the classic "fight-or-flight" response. When life threat becomes overwhelming or inescapable, states of immobilization, collapse, and dissociation are mediated by the dorsal vagal complex.

Polyvagal Theory also brings to light the concept of neuroception, the unconscious process of the continuous appraisal the autonomic nervous system makes of the environment—whether it is safe, dangerous, or life-threatening. This process works below the level of conscious awareness but dramatically influences the emergence of physiological states, emotional experiences, and active behaviors observable at any given moment.

In providing an articulated yet scientifically based conceptual framework for the understanding of the intricate activities of the autonomic nervous system, Polyvagal Theory is a powerful lens into the discoveries and paradigms of the human journey. These have far-reaching implications for our understanding of stress, trauma, emotional regulation, and social connection and, thus, for developing innovative approaches to therapy and practice in cultivating resilience and well-being.

As we journey through the key ideas and applications of the Polyvagal Theory in this chapter, I encourage you to hold the central idea in mind: our autonomic nervous system is a brilliant and adaptive system designed by the forces of evolution to foster survival, connection, and growth. By understanding and working with the wisdom of this system, we can unlock robust pathways to healing, regulation, and thriving.

2.2 The Three Hierarchical Subsystems of the Autonomic Nervous System

At the core of Polyvagal Theory is the appreciation that the autonomic nervous system is not a single system but is organized into three phylogenetically ordered subsystems. Each of these subsystems has its mechanism of adaptive function and set of visceral, motor, and central neural mechanisms through which adaptive strategies are implemented.

For example, consider the ANS the symphony orchestra; its subsystems play distinctive roles to culminate a complex symphony of our life. Three parts of the ANS — just like all the different instruments within a symphony — are confronting each other in perfect coordination to give shape to our responses to the ever-changing demands of our internal and external environments.

According to Porges, the first and most evolutionarily advanced subsystem is the ventral vagal system complexed with the myelinated vagus nerve. Rich in mammals, this complex system supports the rich social behaviors that are the hallmark of our species: facial expression, vocal communication, listening with an active ear, social engagement, and prosodies. On activation, one is left with an experience of safety, connection, and engagement with others.

The second subsystem is the sympathetic branch, often referred to as the "fight-flight" system; its activation readies the organism for action by accelerating heart rate, rate of respiration, and the flow of blood to the muscles. The mobilization response is adaptive in preparing the body for challenge or danger to respond readily in the face of threat.

The third and most primitive is the dorsal vagal complex, associated with the unmyelinated vagus nerve. It is usually called the "immobilizing" or "shutdown" system because it promotes states of immobilization, collapse, and dissociation in the face of overwhelming threat. While this response can be life-saving in situations of extreme danger, chronic activation of the dorsal vagal complex can harm physical and mental health.

According to the Polyvagal Theory, these three subsystems are organized hierarchically, with the ventral vagal complex acting as a "brake" on the sympathetic and dorsal vagal systems. When the environmental cues suggest safety, the ventral vagal complex is functional and maintains a state of quietness, social engagement, and self-regulation. When presented with a challenge to danger, the sympathetic nervous system recruits, which supports states of mobilization or "fight-or-flight."

If the sympathetic state is not adequate for safety or if the threat is too huge, then the control will shift to the dorsal vagal complex, and states of shutdown or even collapse can be created, the so-called "freeze." Therefore, the autonomic nervous system is hierarchically organized, and it becomes paradigmatic to promote states of ventral vagal dominance whenever possible, in which we feel safe, are connected, and can, therefore, coherently deal with the world around us.

The dynamic interplay amongst these three subsystems is fundamental to healthy autonomic regulation and overall well-being. By cultivating practices that support the activity of the ventral vagal complex, we can enhance our capacity for self-regulation and resilience in the face of life's challenges.

2.3 The Ventral Vagal Complex and Social Engagement System

The ventral vagal complex is the most evolutionarily advanced portion of the autonomic nervous system and modulates our physiological states and social behavior. This system, anchored in the myelinated vagus and its branches to the facial, vocal, and middle ear muscles, provides the neural circuitry for the "social engagement system" by Stephen Porges.

Activation of the ventral vagal complex ideally results in states of calmness, openheartedness, and social connectedness. It provides a "vagal break" to the heart, softening cardiac rhythms. Blood pressure and inflammation are likely to decrease, creating a basal physiological state that can be used for growth, restoration, and healing.

However the functions of the ventral vagal complex go beyond mere regulation for physiology. By way of its connections to the muscles of the face, throat, and middle ear, this system makes it possible for us to perform the complex social behaviors that are the hallmarks of mammalian interaction: facial expressions, vocal prosody, and active listening—the process of social engagement and bonding.

The ventral vagal complex is essential in the extent to which it regulates the autonomic nervous system in a general manner. It acts like a brake for the sympathetic nervous system and dorsal vagal complex, enabling states of calm and connection when we sense safety signals around us. The ventral vagal complex will, however, disengage when presented with a challenge or a threat, letting the sympathetic nervous system mobilize the body for action.

One of the most striking functions of the ventral vagal complex is activating the "tend-and-befriend" response, where the body seeks social support and connection in the face of stress. This response often includes the release of oxytocin, generally known as the "bonding hormone," and is considered to have evolved to ensure social safety and survival.

More importantly, perhaps, the ventral vagal complex is the one that serves the purpose of setting up attachment bonds between the infant and a significant caregiver. Physiological and emotional co-regulation within this system becomes the model by which an infant develops security in an attachment figure—a foundation upon which social and emotional functions develop throughout the lifespan.

However, when the ventral vagal complex does not operate well, social and emotional challenges can arise. Individuals with a history of chronic stress, trauma, or attachment breaks have little access to the calming, connecting aspects of this system and, therefore, become hyperaroused, anxious, or socially withdrawn.

Interventions targeting the ventral vagal complex, working from a social-engagement perspective, may exceptionally be helpful here. These could include, for example, deep breathing, vocal toning, exercises to promote facial expressions, and emphasizing solidarity and attunement.

2.4 The Sympathetic Nervous System and Mobilization

The sympathetic nervous system is one of three main subsystems in the autonomic nervous system; it mobilizes the body into action in challenging or threatening circumstances. Commonly referred to as the "fight or flight" system, it works to make those dramatic physiological changes that instantaneously prepare us to face a danger or to run away from it.

When the sympathetic nervous system is aroused, a quantity of physiological changes ensue : increased heart rate and blood pressure, fast and shallow breathing, diversion of blood from the digestive tract to the muscles—preparing the body to fight in an emergency or exit from it. The pupils dilate to let in more light to the eyes, and there is an increased flow of glucose from the liver to the blood, thus providing energy.

Specifically, stress hormones, particularly adrenaline and cortisol, from the adrenal glands bring about these changes. The hormones, coupled with direct neural innervation from the sympathetic nervous system, induce a state of arousal and focus heightened enough that one can effectively respond to potential threats in the environment.

Activation of the sympathetic nervous system can be life-saving under conditions of acute danger, but its chronic or exaggerated activation can be detrimental to both somatic and mental health. The sustained secretion of stress hormones has been associated with medical illnesses in such diverse groups as cardiovascular disease, gastrointestinal disorders, and immune suppression.

It could also gradually foster states of anxiety, hypervigilance, and irritability as the body remains on alert for danger where there is none. In the long run, this heightened state of activity can affect our relationships, work performance, and overall quality of life.

Most importantly, Polyvagal Theory offers a robust framework and way of seeing sympathetic activation within the context of overall health and well-being. Recognizing the adaptive nature of the fight-or-flight response and its potential risks of being chronically activated, we can develop strategies that allow a balanced and resilient autonomic nervous system.

These might include techniques that assist with down-regulating the sympathetic nervous system—deep breathing, progressive muscle relaxation, and mindfulness meditation. In this way, we learn to perceive and regulate our physiological arousal and develop resilience in the face of stress and challenge.

2.5 The Dorsal Vagal Complex and Immobilization

The dorsal vagal complex represents the most primitive subsystem of the autonomic nervous system, comprising the unmyelinated vagus nerve and the immobilization response. This system said to first arise in early vertebrates, is often called the "freeze" or "shutdown" system because it supports states of profound physiological and behavioral inhibition in the face of overwhelming threats.

Activation of the dorsal vagal complex involves various physiological changes initiated to conserve energy and promote survival under extreme conditions. Heart rate and blood pressure drop, digestion is inhibited, and the body can become still and unresponsive. The state of immobilization is often accompanied by feelings of numbness, detachment, or dissociation from one's bodily sensations and emotions.

Although the immobilization response can be life-saving in situations of actual life threat, such as a predatory attack or a natural disaster, chronic or excessive activation of the dorsal vagal complex can negatively affect physical and mental health. When an individual gets stuck in shutdown or collapse, they may experience a range of symptoms ranging from chronic fatigue and digestive problems to compromised immune function.

Activation of the dorsal vagal complex will also likely dramatically impact the individual's capacity for social engagement and emotional regulation. If the body is immobilized, the ventral vagal complex and its corresponding social engagement system will be offline, so that person will find it difficult to reach out to another or, for that matter, even to the self in emotional experience.

This could set up a vicious cycle whereby the lack of social connection and emotional regulation is further consolidating dorsal vagal complex activation, hurling a creature into even greater states of shutdown and collapse. In the long term, this might contribute to the development of depression, anxiety, and post-traumatic stress disorder.

The Polyvagal Theory offers a helpful organizing principle regarding how the dorsal vagal complex supports our health and well-being. With the recognition that the immobilization response is adaptive and understanding its potential risks with chronic activation, ways can be considered to facilitate an autonomic nervous system that is balanced and resilient.

Some include practices that gently titrate a person out of the frozen through grounding techniques, body-based interventions, and trauma-informed yoga. By learning to recognize and modulate our physiological states, we present ourselves with a greater degree of resilience in the face of stress and challenge.

2.6 Neuroception: Assessing Safety and Danger

One of the most critical insights in Polyvagal Theory has to do with something called neuroception: this is the unconscious process by which our autonomic nervous system is constantly looking for cues of safety, danger, and life threat. This continuous, reflexive appraisal of our surroundings is downloaded into our vital regulatory circuits, influencing the way our physiological states, emotional experiences, and behavioral responses are shaped at any given moment.

Neuroception is the word for an unconscious, implicit, self-organizing system that takes in and filters sensory input in the same way but is built on the more rapid, primitive, subcortical processing of sensory input, unlike conscious perception. It is in constant operation, surveying both our internal and external environments for cues of safety or danger. This rapid and automatic assessment is mediated by neural circuits within the brainstem and limbic system and has adapted to detect and respond to potential risks in our surroundings.

When our perception recognizes the cue of another's safety—that warm smile, accessible voice, soft touch—it allows our system to fully engage with the ventral vagal complex, specifically the social engagement system. We are physiologically calm and open, able to look around and explore, in the mode of growth-oriented behaviors that are foundational for thriving.

But when perception detects a cue of danger or life threat—a harsh tone of voice, an aggressive posture, or a sudden loud noise—it can rapidly trigger activation of the sympathetic nervous system or, depending on the nature and intensity of the threat, dorsal vagal complex. These states of mobilization or immobilization, although potentially life-saving when engaged in actual emergencies, can also lead to a variety of physical, psychological, and social problems when they are chronically or developmentally dysregulated.

But one of the chief implications of neuroception is that our experiences of subjective safety and threat are often at variance with the objective facts of our environment. Thus, for example, this could characterize the state of an individual with a history of trauma or chronic stress, whose perception is highly sensitized to features of danger, even if objectively safe. This can lead to a broad array of problems and hypervigilance, anxiety, and social withdrawal because the autonomic nervous system remains vigilant in preparation for a threat—real or not.

The theory suggests that understanding and working with the process of neuroception is key to promoting resilience, regulation, and well-being. One learns to recognize and modulate their physiological states, hence becoming flexible and very adaptive under stress and challenge.

This can involve practices that help to down-regulate the sympathetic nervous system and support the activation of the ventral vagal complex, like deep breathing, mindfulness meditation, and social engagement exercises. We can help to recalibrate perception by cultivating a sense of inner safety and connectedness that promotes a more balanced, resilient autonomic nervous system.

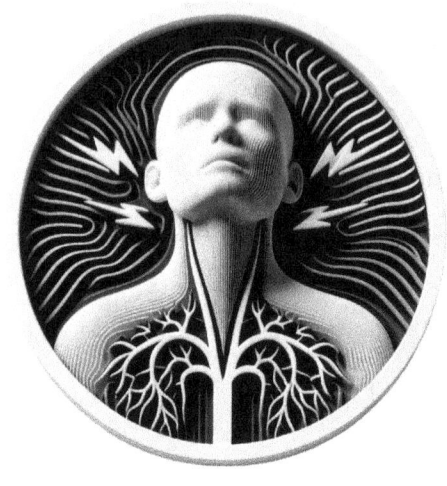

Chapter 3
The Vagus Nerve's Role in Anxiety, Trauma, and Stress

Anxiety, trauma, and chronic stress are the challenges most people will face in their lifetime. Such experiences can leave deeper scars in our psyches and, therefore, profoundly affect our quality of life. However, the vagus nerve has been observed to have a vital role in shaping the emotional landscape and resilience in people facing adversity.

Our chapter will delve more into the exciting interconnections of the vagus nerve with mental health: how this fantastic system mediates, underwrites, and orchestrates experiences of anxiety, trauma, and stress; how these are mechanistically wrought in the physiology of the body; and the new treatment strategies targeting the vagal system in the promotion of emotional homeostasis and resilience.

We will provide practical exercises and the application of these strategies so that you, too, can develop a more resilient and flexible vagus nerve. By the end of the chapter, you will have a much richer understanding of the role of the vagus nerve in your emotional life and a toolkit of practices that support your journey to a life that is more balanced and resilient.

3.1 Anxiety and Vagus Nerve: A Bidirectional Relationship

Anxiety is a common human experience that drives an essential vital function important throughout evolution: to keep us safe in the face of perceived threats. However, if anxiety proves to be chronic, excessive, and not proportionate to the challenges of life, it can then develop into a crippling condition that undermines well-being and functioning.

Recent research has revealed the critical role that the vagus nerve plays in shaping how we experience anxiety. The vagus nerve is critically involved in the system of stress response in the body, balancing regeneration and, through its primary system, reconciling the branches of the autonomic nervous system—the sympathetic and the parasympathetic.

In the presence of an optimally functioning vagus, this will allow the possibility of "braking" the responses to stress and the return to feelings of quiet safety and social interaction. With low vagal tone, the sympathetic nervous system may become overactive, leading to rising levels of chronic anxiety, hypervigilance, and emotional dysregulation.

All this is evident from various physical and psychological symptoms, such as muscle tension, pounding of the heart, shallow breathing, significant worry, and concentration or relaxation problems. Long-term anxiety can take a heavy toll on physical and mental well-being in the form of heart diseases, gastrointestinal disorders, and depression.

Thankfully, an expanding range of studies indicate that vagal-targeted interventions are, in fact a very potent form of treatment for anxiety. Deep diaphragmatic breathing, mindfulness meditation, chanting – many of these practices that have been found to stimulate the vagus nerve have physiological calm and emotional balance as their outcome effects.

By cultivating a more vital, more resilient vagus nerve, we can also develop a more remarkable ability to handle life's ups and downs with ease and equanimity. The following sections will outline many concrete strategies and exercises that you can use to harness the power of your vagus nerve in the service of your anxiety management and well-being.

3.2 Effects of Trauma on the Vagus Nerve and Autonomic Regulation

Trauma, which can be either experienced from a one-time overwhelming event or chronic inescapable stress, leaves a mark on the nervous system. What this means is that, for numerous trauma survivors, their body's natural stress response disregulates, giving way to a collection of physical, emotional, and cognitive challenges that usually persist well past the point when the threat has disappeared.

A primary conduit through which this dysregulation occurs is the impact of trauma on the functioning of the vagus nerve in autonomic regulation. When a massive threat is engaged, the body's response for survival proceeds under the direction of the autonomic nervous system, which has two branches: the sympathetic "fight-or-flight" and the parasympathetic "rest-and-digest" branches.

Ideally, in a healthy nervous system, these two branches work in dynamic balance with each other, with the vagus nerve acting as the central brake. However, under conditions of extreme or prolonged stress, this balance can fall apart. The sympathetic branch may become chronically overactivated, leading to states of hyperarousal. In contrast, the vagally mediated parasympathetic branch may become suppressed, denying the body the ability to return to a state of calm or restoration.

This dysregulation can manifest in a range of symptoms often associated with post-traumatic stress disorder (PTSD), such as hypervigilance, intrusive memories, emotional numbness, and sleep disturbances. For many trauma survivors, a stuck autonomic nervous system keeps them locked into a fight-or-flight arousal pattern or shut down in collapse.

The insights of polyvagal theory by Dr. Stephen Porges provide a window through which to understand and treat the nervous system's response to trauma. Highlights here include the critical role of the vagus in mediating safety and social engagement and strategies toward promoting vagal regulation and resilience.

Interventions with the vagus nerve, such as Somatic Experiencing, Sensorimotor Psychotherapy, and EMDR, have been very hopeful for their potential to assist trauma survivors in recentering and establishing a greater sense of embodied safety and security through the autonomic nervous system. Working directly with the body's survival responses and encouraging vagal engagement enables one to transcend the cycles of hyperarousal and dissociation, leading to eventual integration and resilience.

In the following few sections, we will explore specific practices and exercises that can help support vagal regulation and nervous system healing in the context of trauma recovery. One can develop an understanding of the vagus nerve's role in both trauma and resilience, helping them empower self and the other with compassion, wisdom, and skill in the healing journey.

3.3 Chronic Stress, Resilience, and the Vagus Nerve

Chronic stress is one of the most pressing challenges of this current time in a constantly moving world, impacting all. Unlike acute stress—another form that is a normal, adaptive response to challenges—chronic stress arises from the long-term perception of either losing control over challenging situations or an overwhelming amount of pressure. With the time and persistent strain that a person faces, digs deep furrows into the health of body and mind, reduces resilience in people, and makes the quality of their lives poor.

The vagus nerve is central to the body's stress-response system and, in a significant way, an essential mediator of the delicate balance within the autonomic nervous system between sympathetic activation and parasympathetic relaxation. A healthy vagus will act almost like a natural brake against stress—down-regulating arousal and fostering calm, safety, and social engagement.

In chronic stress conditions, however, the delicate balance of the autonomic nervous system may be upset. The fight-or-flight sympathetic branch may become chronically overactivated and, thus, be responsible for the development of states of hypervigilance, anxiety, and even inflammation. Meanwhile, the parasympathetic "rest and digest" branch, mediated via the vagus nerve, may become suppressed, impairing the body's capacity for recovery and restoration.

This may bring about various physical and psychological symptoms, such as chronic muscle tension, problems of the digestive tract, sleep, mood, and concentration disturbances. Over the long term, continuous stress can be at the root of serious health issues, including heart diseases, autoimmune disorders, and mental health disorders like depression and anxiety.

Building resilience to face chronic stress, therefore, requires a multifactorial approach that appreciates not only the external sources of stressful stimuli but also the internal capacity for self-regulation. Central to this process is the support for health and tone in the vagus nerve, which is critical in moderating stress reactivity and fostering physiological and emotional balance.

It has been proven that techniques such as deep-diaphragmatic breathing, chanting, and cold water immersion that stimulate the vagus nerve are compelling ways of reducing stress and building resilience. Done regularly, they help strengthen our "vagal brake" and improve our ability to down-regulate stress, thereby developing resilience in being calm and focused in the face of challenges.

In addition to the specific vagus nerve exercises mentioned above, resilience can be fostered even further by working with lifestyle factors that may help or harm vagal tone: adequate sleep, regular movement, nutrient-dense nutrition, and the wholeness of positive social connectedness.

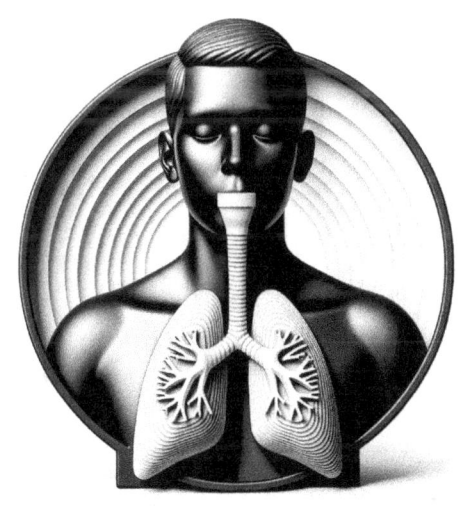

Chapter 4
Breathing Exercises to Stimulate the Vagus Nerve

In this fast world, one will easily get overwhelmed, stressed, and out of touch with oneself. But what if I told you that there is one very potent tool that can be used to negotiate these challenges with more ease and greater resilience? It is a tool you are born with, which is always available to you, and it is free—it is your breath.

In the remainder of this chapter, you'll continue to learn a variety of exercises in breathing that will help stimulate this excellent vagus nerve—the master of the parasympathetic nervous system. Through conscious breathing, we've got the power to activate the body's natural relaxation response, allowing one to emotionally feel good, experience a more profound sense of inner peace, and feel alive.

Whether you are a novice or an experienced breathworker, you will find the practices outlined in this chapter to offer an extensive toolkit of resources to support you in your journey towards more health, happiness, and resilience. So, take a deep breath, and let's dive in.

4.1 Diaphragmatic Breathing: The Foundation of Vagal Tone

Central to any effective breathing exercise is diaphragmatic breathing. This exercise is also sometimes called belly breathing or deep breathing, which involves the full engagement of the diaphragm, a dome-shaped muscle located right at the base of the lungs. During inhalation, the diaphragm contracts and flattens, enabling more space for the lungs to expand and draw in air. Then, during exhalation, the diaphragm will always be seen to relax and rise, thus enabling the lungs to expel air.

Unfortunately, most of us have gotten into a lifetime habit of this shallow, chest-breathing process, which is a contributing factor to a wide range of health problems, such as anxiety, muscle tension, and fatigue. Learning to breathe with our diaphragm allows access to this powerful way of being able to stay relaxed and reduce the stress level many times over.

The benefits and the healthy effects of diaphragmatic breathing are numerous and have far-reaching outcomes. Research has shown that routine practice can:

1. Activates the parasympathetic nervous system - reduces stress and anxiety

2. Enhances HRV, a biomarker for vagal tone, and hence resilience.

3. Enhances mental clarity and focus, as much oxygen will be pumped to the brain.

4. Improves the quality of sleep and helps reduce insomnia

5. Reducing chronic pain by releasing muscle tension and inducing a state of relaxation.

Diaphragmatic breathing can be practiced in a seated position or lying down comfortably, with one hand placed on your chest and the other on your belly. Breathe slowly and mindfully through your nose, expanding your belly so that the hand on your stomach rises while keeping the hand on your chest relatively still. Out through pursed lips, noticing your belly fall. Continue smooth, deep, and even breaths in a slow, rhythmic pattern.

Make diaphragmatic breathing part of your life by doing it consistently. In a way, this will help empower you toward better and improved levels of health and well-being. By putting this foundational technique into your life, you will be considerably closer to making your vagal tone stronger and more resilient.

4.2 Box Breathing: A Tool to Calm and Focus

Most of all, in those highly stressful, overwhelming moments, or really during any kind of super intense feeling, a quick but effective way to just get back to peace and clarity can make all the difference in the world. And that is where a simple, powerful technique like box breathing comes into play.

Box breathing is the process in which one breathes in, holds the breath, and exhales for equal counts; this provides symmetry and a sense of balance through the movements of the breath. With a constructed rhythm, focus can be drawn from breath to mind in calming, quieting, reducing stress, and producing an inner awake state of peacefulness.

The technique is straightforward:

1. Take a slow, deep breath through your nose for a count of four, filling your lungs from the bottom to the top.

2. Hold your breath for a count of four, allowing your body to be still.

3. Exhale through your mouth slowly to the count of four, emptying your lungs completely.

4. Retain the breath for a further count of four before inhaling the next breath.

Stop and start this cycle a few minutes at a time while maintaining an even and steadier pace during the drill.

The physiological benefits of box breathing are related to its power in regulating the autonomic nervous system. Through an activation of the parasympathetic response, this practice can bring down the heart rate, lower blood pressure, and bestow a sense of calm and relaxation. At the same time, due to the very nature of the technique being focused, it can significantly enhance mental clarity, concentration, and performance under pressure.

Olivia was an executive with a hectic schedule, suffering from a considerable amount of work-related stress. She found that by sparing just a few minutes each day for practicing box breathing, this activity improved her anxiety levels and her ability to handle situations more efficiently and calmly.

Incorporating box breathing into your day can be as easy as putting three minutes aside in the morning or evening to practice or using it whenever you need a short reset during tension or after transitions. With consistent practice, this powerful technique can become a reliable ally in your quest for greater peace, focus, and resilience.

Alternate Nostril Breathing: Balancing the Body and Mind

Nadi Shodhana, or alternate nostril breathing, is understood to be one of the most potent practices for balance, harmony, and overall well-being in the web of yogic practices. Rooted in the ancient Indian wisdom traditions, it is a pattern of specific breathing through one nostril at a time, creating a sense of equilibrium and calm.

According to the philosophy of yoga, the body is crisscrossed by a vast network of energy channels known as nadis, through which prana—the vital force—circulates. Two principal nadis responsible for these circulations are the idea, to the left side of the spine, and Pingala, to the right. Ida represents the qualities of coolness, calmness, and introspective nature, while Pingala represents heat, energy, and extroversion.

By changing the flow of breath between these two channels, alternate nostril breathing is brought to balance and creates harmony in the energetic system of the body, which allows the individual to experience a sense of physical, mental, and emotional well-being. Studies have shown that regular practice can lead to a range of benefits, including:

1. Reduced stress and anxiety

2. Improved cardiovascular function and lung capacity.

3. Improved mental clarity and increased focus

4. Improves quality of sleep; reduces insomnia

5. Enhanced emotional regulation and resilience.

To practice Alternate Nostril Breathing, assume a comfortable seated position with the spine erect and shoulders relaxed. With your right hand, fold your index and middle fingers into your palm so that your thumb, ring finger, and pinky are extended toward your nose. Then close your right nostril with your thumb and inhale deeply through your left nostril. Exhale through the right nostril, then inhale and exhale through the left nostril. Inhale through the right nostril again, then close it with the thumb and exhale through the left. This is one complete cycle. Continue in this pattern with your breath steady and even.

As you practice, you may notice a growing sense of calm, balance, and inner stillness. With regular practice, alternate nostril breathing can become a powerful tool for navigating life's challenges with greater equanimity and grace.

Hannah was a college student who had been suffering from problems related to anxiety and lack of sleep. She finally found some relief in the breathing practice of an alternate nostril. With this practice integrated into her life, she almost immediately saw changes in her sleeping patterns and her ability to manage stress and emotions. Alternate nostril breathing was the doorway to intense self-awareness and calmness for Hannah.

Whether you are a seasoned yogi or new to the path of breathwork, alternate nostril breathing is one of the simplest and most profound ways to bring about balance and resilience in one's life. Use this wisdom of an ancient practice and walk away with the tool to better wade through the ebbs and flows of modern life.

4.4 The 4-7-8 Breathing Technique: A Natural Tranquilizer

In this rapidly moving and somewhat annoying world, one could consider the power of a straightforward and effective way to quiet the mind and relax the body as a real blessing. Enter the 4-7-8 breathing technique. It has been called a "natural tranquilizer" because it brings about a powerful relaxation effect on the body by effectively reducing stress and anxiety.

The 4-7-8 breathing technique adheres to a pattern set up by the same renowned Dr. Andrew Weil, a pioneer in integrative medicine, on the model of pranayama—the ancient yoga breathing practice. It is said to help calm the nervous system, reduce stress, and bring inner peace and well-being through a specific rhythm of inhaling, holding, and exhaling.

The technique is simple yet powerful:

1. Exhale with your whole body, releasing the whooshing sound through your mouth.

2. With your mouth closed, breathe silently through your nose to a count of four.

3. Take a deep breath and hold it for a count of seven.

4. Breathe out entirely through your mouth, making a whoosh sound to a count of eight.

5. Repeat this process so that in the end, you have taken four breaths.

The 4-7-8 breathing technique works by utilizing the parasympathetic nervous system that causes the "rest and digest" response of the body. By extending the exhale and slowing the breath, the technique helps to work against the effects of the sympathetic nervous system, which may be further inflected by stress and anxiety.

Regular practice of the 4-7-8 breathing technique yields multiple benefits:

1. Reduces stress and anxiety

2. Better sleep with less trouble falling asleep

3. Blood pressure and heart rate decreased

4. Increased mental clarity and focus

5. Increased emotional regulation and resilience

The 4-7-8 breathing technique was a miracle of saving grace to Ethan, a young professional who had been ridden by stress and anxiety emanating from his work. Spending just a few minutes each day practicing this deceptively simple but powerful exercise, he had been able to cut his stress levels in half and acquire much more inner peace and clarity. This made the 4-7-8 breathing technique an essential tool for Ethan to help him navigate the many challenges of his professional busyness with a little less effort and resilience.

It doesn't take much to work the 4-7-8 breathing technique into your life: in the morning, in the evening, or simply take a few minutes out of a busy schedule. This powerful technique, through continued practice, becomes like an old friend—a reliable ally in your quest for greater peace, well-being, and resilience in the face of life's challenges.

4.5 Ujjayi Breathing: The Breath of Victorious Warrior

Among the rich and varied landscape of yogic practices, Ujjayi breathing shines as a jewel, a technique so unique that it can transform the body, mind, and spirit. It is also referred to as the "breath of the victorious warrior" or "ocean breath." Ujjayi involves a specific process of conscious breathing accompanied by a soft, audible sound, like the rhythmic murmur of waves breaking upon a distant shore.

Ujjayi breathing is the breathing pretty much synonymous with strength, power, and graceful poise under duress. Like a skillful warrior who, even in the heat of battle, never loses his center and focus, the practitioner of Ujjayi learns how to maintain calm and centered in the face of life's challenges.

Ujjayi breath: Begin by finding a comfortable seated position, with a straight back but a relaxed body. Close the mouth and breathe in and out through the nose. Now, simply notice the breath as it travels in and out. Practice the last breath as though you were fogging up a mirror. With that breath, you slightly constrict the muscles in the base of your throat. This constriction should create a sound similar to the ocean's distant roar.

Try to maintain this slight stricture and the sound of your breath even on both the inhalation and the exhalation, allowing your breath to find a smooth, even rhythm. Keep working that way for a few minutes, settling your mind in and holding the texture of the Ujjayi breath.

A key advantage of Ujjayi breathing is its profound quality of calming the nervous system. The slow and steady rhythm of the breath, along with its hypnotic sound, activates the parasympathetic nervous system to bring about deep relaxation and ease.

The breath equally becomes a potent tool in cultivating presence and mindfulness. It takes all of our attention to the subtleties of the breath. With that, the mind will settle, dissolve distractions, and we are more fully present in the here and now. From that eye in the center of the Ujjayi storm, we can face life's challenges with much more clarity, resilience, and grace.

Sarah, on the other hand, is a working mother of two; the Ujjayi breathing was her lifeline for a particularly stressful period in her life. She said that with this practice included in her daily yoga routine, she just felt a significant difference in being able to cope with stress, usually in sustaining an attitude of inner calm amidst the chaos of family life. Thus, Ujjayi breathing for Sarah became not only part of practice but part of her—a resource to be drawn on at any time to bring more peace, balance, and resilience into life.

Whether you are a seasoned yogi or are new to the practice, Ujjayi breathing offers a powerful portal to a deeper relationship with your breath, your body, and your inner landscape. With patience in practice and loving intention, this ancient technique can become a faithful companion on your journey through life, reminding you at each breath of your innate strength, wisdom, and resilience.

4.6 Breath of Fire: Igniting Vitality and Focus

In the dynamic world of Kundalini Yoga, Breath of Fire is an extraordinary tool that vivifies the body, calms the mind, and wakes up the nervous system. It is a type of fast, rhythmic, and controlled raise of the active exhalation and passive inhalation of breath, acting as a natural stimulant of the body in the raising of energy levels and awakening of the body and mind.

To do Breath of Fire, sit comfortably and elongate your spine, relaxing the shoulders. Exhale sharply out the nose and pull the navel sharply in and up towards the spine on the exhale. Let the inhale occur passively and naturally as the diaphragm lifts, and the air is naturally sucked back into the lungs. Continue in this pattern, maintaining an approximate 2–3 breaths per second rhythm.

Breath of Fire feels strange, even forced, at first. After a bit of practice, it becomes as natural and effortless as ordinary breathing. As you practice this dynamic breath, you will probably find it comes with an incredible list of powerful benefits, including the following:

1. Increased energy and sense

2. Better clarity of thoughts and focus on

3. Reduces stress and

4. Enhanced lung capacity and improved respiratory function.

5. Increased immunity

6. Enhanced emotional balance and resilience

At the physiological level, the Breath of Fire excites the sympathetic nervous system with an energy boost for feeling alert and awake naturally. Simultaneously, the fast inspiration and expiration involved in the practice will calm the mind and bring you to a state of centered presence to navigate challenges in life with clarity and equanimity.

Michael found the Breath of Fire to be a game-changer for him. Waking up every morning and performing this dynamic practice, he began feeling energized and clear in his mind, with a sense of well-being. The Breath of Fire was just the tool Michael needed at that moment: to fuel his inner fire and walk this life journey with the radiance and resilience he desired.

Whether you are a seasoned yogi or just discovering the power of your breath, the Breath of Fire is a powerful, available way to tune into your core with strength, clarity, and vitality. Practiced consistently and with an open, curious mindset, this powerful technique will, over time become another asset on your journey to more excellent health, happiness, and resilience in all areas of life.

4.7 Bhramari Pranayama: The Humming Bee Breath

In this silent world of yogic breathwork lies Bhramari Pranayama, also known as Humming Bee Breath, a soft, serene practice that carries great strength in calming the mind, reducing stress, and bringing deep inner peace and well-being. Its name is from the Sanskrit word for "bee," and it is a process of making a soft humming sound while exhaling, producing a vibration that is very soothing in the head and chest.

To practice Bhramari Pranayama, do so sitting in a comfortable posture, with closed eyes and a relaxed body. With your index fingers, bring them to exert a little pressure on the ears so the sound from outside is closed off. Now breathe in through your nostrils, taking a deep breath and filling your lungs. Breathe out, making a deep and steady humming sound, just like the gentle buzzing of a bee. Repeat this process for a few breaths, allowing the mind to rest in that comforting resonance of the sound.

The Bhramari Pranayama effects are instant and profound; the soft humming vibration is like the internal massage of the vagus nerve, thus stimulating the parasympathetic nervous system and leading to deep relaxation and calm. Regular practice has shown the following benefits:

1. Reduced stress and anxiety

2. Lowered blood pressure and heart rate

3. Better Quality Sleep and Cure for Insomnia

4. Better mental clarity and focus

5. Emotional self-regulation and resilience

In a more profound sense, Bhramari Pranayama offers a powerful tool to develop mindfulness and inner awareness. Whenever you direct your attention to those subtle sensations of the humming breath, by it, you are naturally stepping aside from the vicious cycles of ruminative thought and emotional reactivity that most frequently underlie stress and anxiety. This simple yet powerful technique, inculcated regularly, can help one attain a sense of inner serenity, clarity, and strength in the face of adversity.

Emma was a college-going student in the middle of the semester, fighting anxiety and stress. Bhramari Pranayama had become such a boon for her. When she started this gentle practice daily, she found a sudden snowballing of stress and felt a great sense of inner peace or emotional balance. Bhramari Pranayama became the best tool for Emma to sail through the fluctuations, sometimes with ease and sometimes with grace.

Whether you're experienced in practice or relatively new to breathwork, Bhramari Pranayama offers a straightforward yet potent way to tune into the wisdom of your breath and find a more profound sense of inner peace and well-being. This ancient technique becomes a supportive friend on the journey through life, reminding you of your capacities for calm, clarity, and resilience with patient practice and loving intentions, humming with every breath.

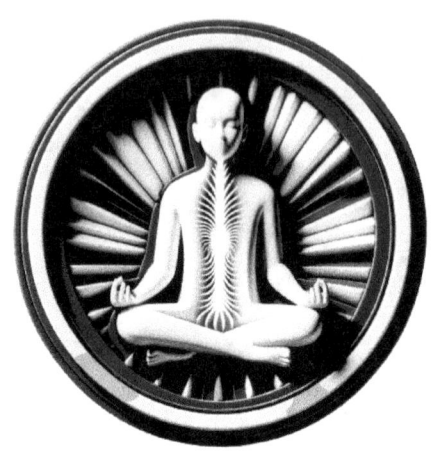

Chapter 5
Mindfulness and Meditation Practices for Vagal Tone

It is almost a fact that stress and anxiety are part of the familiar bedfellows in this fast-paced modern world of ours. We rush through our days with our minds agog, often disconnected from our bodies and the present moment. But what if there was a way to find calm amidst the chaos and make ourselves resilient in life's challenges? Enter the practice of mindfulness and meditation.

Mindfulness, at its very root, is the simple practice of being present and aware in the moment without judgment. By learning to watch our thoughts, emotions, and physical sensations with curiosity and acceptance, we break free from that pattern of stress and reactivity.

About deep relaxation and inner peace, it is meditation is a close ally of mindfulness. Techniques range from following one's breath to visualizing peaceful scenes, like various techniques of meditation that could draw us into an experience of profound rest and alertness.

And more than mere aids to relaxation, mindfulness and meditative states themselves are now under the microscope for their transformational effects –literally: On the physical and psychological well-being of those who enter them. An increasing number of scientific studies indicate that regular mindfulness and meditation reduce stress and anxiety, improve emotional regulation, boost immune function, and change the brain to promote greater resilience.

Auspicious are the effects of mindfulness and meditation on the vagus nerve, an essential component of the parasympathetic nervous system. This nerve applies a brake to the stress reaction and, thereby, promotes bodily activities for rest and digestion. We tone our vagus nerve through mindfulness and meditation, and we get a more balanced and resilient nervous system in return.

This chapter includes mindfulness and meditation practices to support vagal tone and overall well-being. From the tools for foundational practices—breath awareness and body scans—to more advanced practices like loving-kindness meditation and Transcendental Meditation, this chapter is an excellent storehouse of resources to support one in navigating more of life's stresses from a place of ease and equanimity.

5.1 Breath Awareness and Loving-Kindness Meditation

The simplest breath is the most powerful tool for the practice of mindfulness. Our breath never leaves us; it is an anchor to the present moment. By learning to tune into the rhythm of our in-breaths and out-breaths, we can cultivate a deep sense of calm and centeredness.

Breath awareness meditation is simple and involves a natural flow of breathing without trying to change or control it. Here is a step-by-step guide:

1. Be seated in a place where you will not be bothered. You can sit on a cushion, yoga pad, or chair with your feet flat on the ground.

2. Gently close your eyes or leave them softly focused on a point before you.

3. Begin with some deep breaths, allowing your abdomen to rise with each inhalation and fall very slightly with each exhalation.

4. Now, leave your breath to its natural rhythm. Just watch that breath is going in and out of the nostrils or observe the calmness of the rise and fall of the chest or belly.

5. Whenever you realize your mind has wandered (as it will), gently release the thought and carry your attention back to the breath. There is no need to judge or berate yourself—noticing and coming back is the practice.

6. This can be continued for 5–10 minutes or as long as you wish. When you are ready, slowly and gently open your eyes. Pause for a moment to feel what it is like to have your eyes open.

If you include this in your daily routine, you will probably realize that the level of ease and presence unfolding is newly possible both within and extending far beyond the meditation practice itself. You are training your mind to be more focused and less reactive, a skill that may profoundly influence your relationship to stress and challenge.

Loving-Kindness Meditation

Breath awareness, in turn, is the basis of mindfulness practice; loving-kindness meditation, or metta, cultivates heart qualities—like compassion, empathy, and unconditional positive regard.

The practice involves repeating phrases expressing goodwill, first toward oneself and then increasingly toward others. By consciously evoking feelings of love and kindness, we begin to soften the boundaries that separate self from others, replacing judgment and aversion with acceptance and care.

Here's how to practice loving-kindness meditation:

1. Find a quiet place and sit comfortably, just as in breath awareness meditation. Close your eyes or keep a soft gaze.

2. Begin by taking a few deep breaths, grounding yourself in the present moment.

3. Now, silently recite the following phrases to yourself, focusing on

feelings of warmth and kindness:

- May I be happy
- May I be healthy
- May I be safe
- May I live with ease

4. After a few minutes, expand your well-wishes to include a loved one, picturing them in your mind as you recite:

- May you be happy
- May you be healthy
- May you be safe
- May you live with ease

5. Next, extend your loving-kindness to a neutral person, someone you neither strongly like nor dislike. Repeat the phrases with this person in mind.

6. Now comes the challenging part - directing loving-kindness toward a difficult person, someone who has caused you pain or with whom you currently experience tension. See if you can wish them well, just as you have for yourself and others.

7. Finally, radiate loving-kindness outward to all beings, without exception:

- May all beings be happy

- May all beings be healthy

- May all beings be safe

- May all beings live with ease

8. When you're ready, gently open your eyes and take a moment to notice how you feel.

This can be clumsy at first, perhaps even seeming a little fake at times, especially with so many of the phrases directing kindness toward yourself or toward that problematic person. But with repetition and practice, you may notice a genuine softening and opening of your heart. You're retraining your mind to incline toward kindness rather than judgment, toward connection rather than separation.

This simple shift can have profound ripple effects in your life regarding your emotional well-being and the general quality of your relationships. When cultivating loving-kindness, you also contribute to a more compassionate world, starting with the most fundamental relationship—that with yourself.

Integrating the Breath and Loving-Kind

As you become more advanced, this next suggested pairing with Metta practice can be pretty potent. There's a way to integrate the two:

1. Start with a few minutes of breath awareness, feeling presence.

2. With each in-breath, say to yourself, "May I be happy, may I be healthy."

3. With each outbreath, say to yourself quietly, in your mind: "May I be safe, may I live with ease."

4. After a few minutes, bring to mind, alternately, a loved one, then a neutral person, then a difficult person, and finally all being, repeating the phrases so they are in sync with the in-and-out-breath.

5. Conclude with a few minutes of simple breath awareness.

As you anchor the loving-kindness phrases with your breath, you are weaving mindfulness and compassion practices together. It is training your heart to work as one—leading to a more balanced and loving way of being.

Be gentle and kind with yourself in integrating these practices into your daily life. Some days, the mind will be more restless or the heart more resistant, but this is all part of the natural process. The key is to keep showing up with openness and self-compassion.

The more you practice, the more Breath Awareness and Loving Kindness become cherished allies on the path of well-being: reliable sources of calm, clarity, and connection amidst the inevitable ups and downs of life. May these practices serve to nourish and support you on your journey.

5.2 Body Scan and Walking Meditation

During our busy lives, it is frequently straightforward to lose contact with our bodies. We are driven to ignore fatigue, to downplay the indications of tension, and we are so commonly on automatic pilot that we have only a faint notion of the wealth of bodily activity. The fact that you are doing this means that you are actively working against this significant disconnection. It invites you to re-awaken connections to that often overlooked realm of embodied experience.

In a body scan, we systematically guide our attention through the body, from the toes to the crown, noticing what sensations are present with an attitude of curiosity and acceptance. The practice is a way of befriending the body, of learning to listen to its subtle messages and to respond with care and kindness.

This can be a step-by-step guide to doing a body scan practice:

1. Starting in a comfortable lying position, your arms should be at your sides, and your legs straight out. You might want to lay on a mat or blanket for cushioning. If lying down is uncomfortable, you can also practice seated in a chair.

2. Gently close your eyes and take a few deep breaths as you feel the body settling into the surface beneath you.

3. Become aware now of sensations occurring in the toes of your left foot—tingling, warmth, pressure, or nothing in particular. Notice whatever sensory experiences may be taking place in the toes. Again, without evaluating or trying to change the experience, just

becoming aware of it through the gentle curiosity of the mind.

4. Slowly raise your attention upward to the sole, then the heel, the top side of the foot, and then the ankle. Each time, pause for a moment and notice sensations with interest and friendliness.

5. Continue this process of scanning slowly up through the body—to the calf, knee, thigh, hip, and pelvis; the belly, chest, and back; the fingers, hands, wrists, forearms, elbows, upper arms, and shoulders; the neck, face, and finally the crown of the head.

6. L et awareness widens so you may feel the whole body; sense the in and out-breath through the entire body. Let it be like this for a few moments.

7. To end the session, wiggle your fingers and toes and then take another deeper breath in. And whenever you feel ready, slowly open your eyes.

As you practice the body scan, you are training the mind to be in the present, ever more attentive to your bodily experience. You are developing a quality of inner listening, an openness to whatever wisdom the body offers. That sometimes leads to a felt sense of embodiment, of inhabiting the body entirely.

It will be very typical to have feelings of restlessness, sleepiness, and frustration during the body scan, especially at the beginning of the practice. The mind may wander incessantly or certain parts of the body seem numb or unreachable. All of this is normal; the important thing is to face whatever comes up with patience and non-judgment and possibly to guide the attention back to the body, time and time again.

Over time and with regular practice, you may also notice more subtlety in physical sensations and an enhanced capacity to be with discomfort or intensity. You may also find that the body scan starts to infiltrate your daily life with more mindfulness during day-to-day activities, such as walking, eating, or even brushing your teeth.

The body scan is an invitation, in a way, to befriend the body—treat it with kindness and attention, which it merits. In a culture that so often pushes against our boundaries or requests that we are in control of the body as an object, this practice is an act of self-care strong enough to transform us totally in our relationship to stress, pain, and health.

How to Emphasize

Though in most meditation practices, one is generally in a still position, walking meditation is moving mindful; in this practice, we make walking the object of our attention and cultivate a sense of being in the body with each step taken.

Walking meditation may be pretty helpful at those times when the body is restless or when the mind is particularly active. The use of the body in gentle movement helps to anchor the mind into physical sensation, making it easier to keep the focus on the present moment.

This is a simple way to practice walking meditation:

1. Find a quiet space where you can walk comfortably back and forth, either indoors or outside. The path need not be extended.

A simple 10 or 15 feet will be enough.

2. Stand at one end of your path, feet parallel and hip-width apart. Allow yourself a moment to feel the body standing upright—the contact of your feet with the ground.

3. When you feel ready, walk at a natural, purposefully slow pace. At every step, be mindful of walking—the sensation of the foot lifting, the sensation of the foot placing itself back down, the movement of the leg, the shifting of weight.

4. Walk until you reach the end of the path. For just a moment, pause, then really consciously turn around and walk back to the start, with the attention back on the bodily sensations.

5. Keep walking back and forth for the rest of your practice, staying present in the physical experience of walking.

6. Every time the mind does begin to wander off (which, by nature, it likely will), bring it back, gently, to the feelings of the body in movement.

7. To finish the practice, bring it to a close in standing, coming to a pause. Just pause and sense that here is the body, still upright, the breath flowing. And then, in your own time, prepare to change your activity.

Similar to the body scan, walking meditation is not something performed to get somewhere else, nor is it an activity to tick off of the list, but instead it is the event of being along each step of the way. It is the practice of employing the qualities attributed to mindfulness in an activity we regularly perform, becoming automatized and, thus, discovering richness and fullness in an existentially significant experience of every moment.

For a walking meditation, you can go at whatever pace you feel comfortable with, whether that be slow, medium, or fast. You might even experiment with varying the pace, using the speed of walking as an additional object of attention.

Over time, maybe you realize that the mindfulness developed in walking meditation starts to pervade other quarters of your life. You may recognize that you are now more present while walking to work or more attuned to your body during exercise. You're training the mind to be more awake and aware, more in touch with the vitality of the present moment.

Doing a Body Scan and Walking Meditation

The two practices of body scan and walking meditation can support and enrich each other. This is a possibility of one way to work with the two practices' integration:

1. Commence with a small body awareness activity—for example, lying down for 10 to 15 minutes— to help ground the activity of the mind. This will help in the establishment of a baseline awareness of the body.

2. Carefully stand up, with the feeling of the body being balanced upright.

3. Start walking meditation, bringing the same mindfulness devel-

oped in the body scan into the activity of walking. If your mind drifts, you again use the sensations as a bridge back to the present; you may do this just the same as in the sections of the body scan.

4. After completing the walking time, stop already. Take a few extra moments to go through the body again – are there changes in the sensations or the overall mood?

5. Deliberately move on to the next thing you need to do throughout the day while bringing with you the energy of that quality of mindful embodiment.

By combining these practices, you are working to strengthen the mindfulness muscle from different angles; you are training the mind to be present and attentive whether the body is still or in movement.

As you explore these embodied practices, please do so with patience, openness, and self-compassion. The goal here is not to reach some particular state, nor even to banish all thoughts for that matter, but to create a new relationship with one's experience of embodiment—a relationship, hopefully, marked by presence, curiosity, and kindness.

5.3 Mindfulness-Based Stress Reduction and Transcendental Meditation

In the late 1970s, Dr. Jon Kabat-Zinn founded the first-ever program in the same category, Mindfulness-Based Stress Reduction (MBSR), at the University of Massachusetts Medical Center. He believed that ancient knowledge of mindfulness should be integrated with modern science and empirically developed into a practical approach to stress management and fostering one's well-being.

Essentially, MBSR is an 8-week-long intensive program that trains participants to relate differently to stress and challenges in life through mindfulness. The training developed through meditation, body awareness, and mindful movement is geared to cultivate non-judgmental, moment-to-moment awareness. It is a skill that can profoundly change a person's relationship with stress, pain, and illness.

The key components of MBSR are:

1. Formal mindfulness practices: The activities here are body scan meditation, sitting meditation, and gentle yoga. The participants commit to practice these skills for 45-60 minutes daily and six times per week.

2. Didactic material: Information about stress physiology and mindfulness is conveyed through lecture, discussion, and exercises.

3. Group dialogue: The program process is not usually carried out individually; it offers the opportunity for participants to be in a group to share experiences and learn from one another. Such an opportunity provides an enabling environment that successful programs exhibit.

4. Daily Life: Besides the formal practice, participants are encouraged to apply mindfulness to everyday living—like mindful eat-

ing, mindful communication, and using the 3-Minute Breathing Space for mini-meditations in challenging moments.

The efficacy of MBSR has seen corroborated evidence through empirical studies. It has been found that a participant can:

- Lower stress, anxiety and depression
- Progress in choric pain management
- Improving immunity
- Enhanced emotional regulation and resilience
- Positive changes in the structure and function of the brain

These benefits seem to arise from how mindfulness practice reshapes our relationship to stress and difficulty. By learning to observe stressful thoughts, emotions, and sensations with curiosity and non-judgment, we create a bit of space around them—a skill known as decentering. This way, we can react more skillfully to life's challenges without getting pulled into cycles of reactivity and rumination.

MBSR has also been demonstrated to exert therapeutic effects on the autonomic nervous system relative to the functioning of the vagus nerve. In that sense, mindfulness practice works in toning the vagus nerve, such that it cultivates a state of embodied awareness coupled with relaxation and builds our capacity for stress resilience and emotional balance.

Though MBSR is commonly taught in an 8-week format, its core principles and practices can pragmatically be adapted so that they become accessible to almost any person's lifestyle. Indeed, most report that just a few minutes of mindfulness practice added to their daily routine changed their overall sense of well-being and stress levels.

Whether you are working with chronic stress, pain, or illness, or just the hard knocks of daily life, MBSR offers a path toward greater ease, resiliency, and well-being. We learn to be present with whatever is happening in the moment and, in so doing, discover our natural healing and transformative capacities.

Transcendental Meditation

The most widely practiced type of mantra meditation is Transcendental Meditation (TM), introduced to the public in the late 1950s by Maharishi Mahesh Yogi. Unlike mindfulness-based practices, which a focus on awareness of the present moment, TM is the silent repeating of a personal mantra, allowing one to transcend the ordinary thinking process and access a state of deep relaxation and inner calm.

TM is an easy and systematic practice:

1. Sit comfortably, close your eyes.

2. Repeating a personal mantra (a sound or phrase which a certified TM teacher gives) effortlessly, silently.

3. If thoughts come, please return to the mantra with kindness.

4. Practice for 15-20 minutes, two.

Although relatively simple in practice, the effects of transcendental meditation on mind and body have been the focus of over six hundred scientific studies. Among other things, research has proven that regular practice of TM:

- Relieves stress, anxiety, and depression

- Natural blood thinner, reducing blood pressure and the risk of heart disease

- Develops brain activities and creativity.

- Contributes to self-actualization and personal

One of the distinctive aspects of TM is this deep rest that seems to be invoked. During TM practice, the body enters into a state of deep relaxation: respiration is reduced, cortisol levels drop, and blood flow to all brain parts is increased. The result is a restful alertness that releases deep-rooted stress and fatigue.

Like MBSR, TM has also been found to affect vagal tone and improve autonomic balance positively. Continued practice appears to optimize the inherent relaxation response, thus increasing resilience to stress.

While the exact mechanisms may be different, both MBSR and TM are approaches to well-being via the development of inner harmony and balance. They return us to realizing our natural capacity for healing and growth and provide us with tools to tap these resources.

Including all elements of MBSR and

Though MBSR and TM emerge from different traditions, they share the same orientation toward reducing suffering and maximizing human flourishing. These two forms of practice can be synergistic for many people, complementing and strengthening each other.

Here's an example of how you might integrate MBSR and TM:

1. Establish a daily practice of TM by sitting for 15-20 minutes twice daily. This habituation to regular practice starts the stabilization process for the nervous system and establishes a baseline for inner calm.

2. Supplement your practice of TM with mindfulness-based stress reduction techniques, such as the body scan, mindful movement, and the 3-minute Breathing Space. In learning to attend to experience with acceptance, non-judgment, and openness, these practices develop moment-to-moment awareness and the capacity to.

3. Participate in an 8-week MBSR program; if possible, this will get you deeper into the experience of mindfulness practice and provide you with the support of a group practice environment.

4. Bring the principles of mindfulness and transcendence into your daily life: Engaged as you are in work, relationships, or leisure activities, try to approach each moment with a little more presence, openness, and equanimity.

Keep in mind that the keyword of any practice that may be transformative is consistency and patience. Although the benefits of MBSR and TM can be profound, they do cumulatively over time with regular practice. Be gentle with yourself as you incorporate these practices into your life. The path of meditation is not always smooth or linear. There will be days—some of ease and others of difficulty. At such moments, the practice is to meet each instant, each experience, with the same kindness and non-judgment that you cultivate in your formal training.

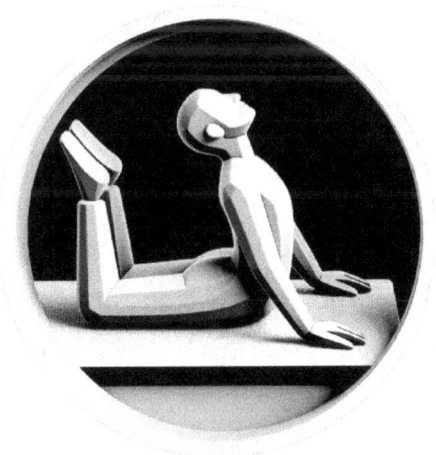

Chapter 6

Yoga Poses and Sequences to Tone the Vagus Nerve

The vagus nerve is the most prolonged and most complex of the 12 pairs of cranial nerves that emerge from the brain. It plays a vital role in the modulation and regulation of all the main bodily functions, which include heart rate, digestion, and metabolism. Doing yoga postures and sequences allows stimulating and exercising this vital nerve with slow, mindful movements and deep breathing. Gentle, restoring practices with breath awareness may facilitate vagal activation, increasing cardiac variability and fostering mental and physical health.

In this yoga program, we balance the calming restorative yoga poses and nourishing yoga sequences with specific instructions to activate your vagus nerve. The restorative poses help the body and mind come anywhere near deep rest and recovery. The sequences encourage the activation of the vagus nerve with structured breath and movement practices designed to ease anxiety and promote alert mind-body awareness.

Feel free to soak in the therapeutic benefits that are felt in the restorative poses. Feel free to experience your body and breath coming to rest. When going through the more active sequences, breathe long and steady, allowing stimulation of the vagus nerve. All this breath-focused, slower-paced practice gives a space for your body's nervous system to take a rest and press reset.

Respect your body and your limitations as you move through your yoga practice. We have shown modifications and alternatives throughout this program to make the practices possible for a broader audience. Just go at your own pace and let your practice unfold however your body resonates in that moment of the practice; don't overdo it or push yourself too hard. Let your yoga be a way to cultivate more relaxation, more awareness in your body, and to be more present in every moment with mindfulness.

For it to equip you with an edge to be resting and moving mindfully in support of your body and mind, this yoga program has a very delicate balance. It is in these moments of rest, in these composed, mindful breathing and movement sequences, that you genuinely get the most from your practice. Take your time and feel these therapeutic qualities in this yoga program.

6.1 The Vagus Nerve and the Relaxation Response

Imagine being stuck in traffic en route to an important meeting. Your heart is probably beating out of control, your palms are sweaty, and you're probably thinking about many things. At times like these, it can feel like the stress has flooded your whole being. However, deep inside your body lies one particular pathway to calmness and relaxation: your vagus nerve.

Often nicknamed the "rest and digest" branch, the parasympathetic nervous system (PNS) works to slow the heart rate, relax muscles, and calm the brain. And, of course, the principal conductor of this delightful symphony is the vagus nerve.

The vagus nerve is the longest of the cranial nerves, which, in a way is quite complex, connecting to many organs: the heart, lungs, and digestive tract, among others. It is one of the most critical nerves in the PNS system. Stimulation of this nerve causes the heart to slow down, thereby reducing the blood pressure and prompting relaxation. This is the relaxation response: the deep resting state antagonist to the fight-or-flight stress response.

Yoga is a holistic system that includes breathwork, meditation, and mindfulness practices proven to stimulate the Vagus nerve and enhance Vagal Tone.

Vagal tone is the strength and efficiency of your vagus nerve in relation to the relaxation response. Those with high vagal tone exhibit lower heart rates, better stress resilience, and greater emotional regulation capacity. They have a well-toned "relaxation muscle."

Many studies have reported an increase in vagal tone and elicited relaxation responses with yoga practices:

1. Slow, deep breathing mimics the vagal tone and thus activates the parasympathetic nervous system in slowing the heart rate and reducing blood pressure, calming down the body.

2. Mindful movement through the yoga postures, when in synchronization with breath awareness, works to create ease and relaxation. It is during specific postures—forward folds and inversions—where vagus nerve stimulation is most evident.

3. Meditation increases present-moment awareness and calms the mind by increasing vagal tone and enhancing the relaxation response.

4. Chant-induced vibrations of "Om" stimulate the vagus nerve, resulting in deep relaxation.

Regular practice of yoga can "tone" the vagus so it can be more effective in its action, calling out the relaxation response when it is needed most. There is growing evidence that yoga has a salutary effect on the PNS and vagal tone.

As a past anxiety and chronic stress sufferer, I understand just how hard it can be to find calm in the chaos of life. Yoga taught me how to discover the power of the relaxation response: how to awaken my inner "calm switch" by quieting my mind with mindful breathing, gentle movement, and meditation. Gradually, the sense of peace that washed over me on my mat generalized into the rest of my life, and my resilience to stress grew.

This change occurred gradually over time and practice: with each mindful breath and movement, we rewire our nervous system for greater peace.

If you're interested in putting your vagus nerve to work for you in relaxation, consider a few easy ways to integrate yoga into your routine:

1. Start each morning with a few minutes of deep diaphragmatic breathing, focusing on the rise and fall of your belly with each inhale.

2. Take frequent breaks and stretch or move mindfully. Even simple postures, such as cat-cow or gentle twists, can stimulate the vagus nerve and promote relaxation.

3.Do a little research on restorative poses like Supported Child's Pose and Reclined Bound Angle, both of which are intended to feel very refreshing.

4. Incorporate a few minutes of short meditations into your daily routine. Both Headspace and Calm provide some excellent guided meditations for beginners.

5. Attend a yoga class or workshop to deepen your practice and learn from experienced teachers. Many studios offer classes specifically for stress relief and relaxation.

Remember: consistency is key. Making relaxation practices part of your life gradually builds calm and resilience.

It is a potent reminder of the wisdom of our body: tapping into this through yoga, we can get equanimity and well-being to cope better with the stresses of life. So, next time you get sucked into that stress spiral, stop, take a good deep breath, move in and out of calamity, and let your vagus nerve guide you back to ease.

6.2 Cat-Cow Pose

Think of a cat stretching lazily in the sun, arching its back and moving sinuously. Imagine a cow, standing still and tranquil, slightly dipped in the middle with its belly hanging low. That's Cat-Cow Pose—the smooth movement to rid you of the tension in your back, support posture improvement, and develop a mind-body connection.

Cat-Cow, for transformation, is a great sequence. It is a straightforward sequence that has become the staple of my daily practice to let go of tension, work on better posture, and relate more deeply to my body and breath.

Cat-Cow Pose, also known as Marjayasana-Bitilasana in Sanskrit, is a fundamental exercise in Hatha Yoga with emphasis on asanas and pranayama in uniting the body with the mind through pureness of the body and calming the mind.

The Sanskrit "Marjaryasana" means cat and "asana" means posture, while "Bitilasana" means cow and "asana." This tandem of postures represents a smoothly flowing sequence conveying natural movements.

The Cat-Cow is a more excellent replication than mere physical mimicry of the animals. In yogic philosophy, the cow is the divine mother—nourishment, abundance, unconditional love. The cat is all about grace, flexibility, and adaptability. Embodying these qualities in our practice, on and off the mat, we cultivate balance, harmony, and resilience.

Benefits of Cat-Cow include:

1. Spinal Health and Flexibility: The movement in flow can achieve lubrication of the spinal joints, an increase in blood supply to the intervertebral discs, and stretching of the back, neck, and shoulder muscles. This ensures that the previously mentioned adverse outcomes of a sedentary lifestyle are averted and a healthy, supple spine is maintained.

2. Improved Posture: The gentle arching and rounding of the spine counterbalances the tendency to hunch forward and reduces upper back and neck tension, increases abdominal muscle tone, and encourages shoulder and head alignment in an appropriate position, leading to more optimally upright, balanced posture and decreasing posturally related aches and pains and other problems.

3. Relief of Stress and Relaxation: The gentle, rhythmic movement of the spine soothes the nervous system and, therefore, the anxious mind, reducing the symptoms of anxiety and tension. The coupling of breath and movement is conducive to being in the here and now of awareness, with the effect of mental chatter being diminished and inner peace emerging.

4. Emotional balance and self-awareness: In these transitions between postures, we learn to observe thoughts, feelings, and physical sensations with detachment and curiosity. This self-inquiry further develops insight into our emotional patterns and triggers, fostering clarity, compassion, and resilience in life's challenges.

5. Preparation for Deeper Practice: Cat-Cow prepares a warm-up exercise of the spine and breath, and it does set a stable platform for more demanding asana and sequences in any style of yoga.

Perform Cat-Cow

1. Begin on the hands and knees, with the wrists under the shoulders and the knees under the hips. The toes are tucked under, fingers are spread wide, and there is a firm press into the.

2. Find a neutral spine, flat back, and a soft gaze on the floor ahead.

3. Breathe in, arch back, and lift chest and tailbone to the sky. Shoulders relaxed, gaze soft, belly sinks to the floor. This is Cow Pose (Bitilasana).

4. Exhale, round back, tuck chin to chest, navel to spine. Imagine a string gently pulling the tailbone to the floor, curving the upper back. This is Cat Pose (Marjaryasana).

5. Flow through the sequence smoothly, moving only with inhalation and exhalation. Inhale to Cow Pose, exhale to Cat Pose. Let the breath lead the way through the movements, but.

6. Attention to the sensations in the spine and the tension zones in the spine. Use the breath to soften and release, letting the breath energy flow along the spine.

7. Repeat about 5-10 breaths or more. Come out by lowering the spine back to neutral, resting in the child's pose.

Variations and modifications include:

- Wrist sensitivity: Place a blanket or towel under your palms to reduce the pressure or practice with the forearms on the mat and elbows under your shoulders.

- Neck pain: maintain a slight gaze forward in Cow, and don't lift your chin high. You can always use a blanket or block for your forehead.

- Knee sensitivity: put a blanket or pillow under your knees for padding, or separate your legs to a stance that reduces pressure.

- Seated variation: sitting on the edge of the chair, feet flat, hands on knees. Inhale and arch your back, lifting your chest; exhale and round your back, tuck your chin. Flow with the breath.

- Breath and movement: take a deep breath, arch the back in Cow for a twist right, then exhale to Cat for a twist left. Continue to move in this way, alternating from side to side upon each breath cycle, moving slowly.

Listen to your body and modify as needed in order to find a safe, comfortable, and nourishing practice for you.

Do the Cat-Cow throughout your day in these ways:

- Practice in bed or on a mat as a morning wake-up to awaken the spine, stimulate circulation, and set a positive tone for the day.

- During workday breaks, to help reduce back, neck, and shoulder tension, minimize eye strain, and improve posture and increase energy and focus.

- As an evening wind-down to de-stress the day, calm the nervous system, and prepare for restful sleep.

- Interposed between other poses as a transition to pause, reconnect with breath, and move with intention and awareness.

Consistency is key. Just a couple of minutes per day of practicing Cat-Cow can have a profound, healthy physical and emotional effect over time.

General FAQs:

1. Do I need to be flexible to practice yoga? No, yoga is not about achieving a pretzel shape but rather mindful movement and breath, meeting your body where it is with acceptance and compassion.

2. How many times should I practice to have effects? Practicing many times is good; however, it is best to develop this into a regular activity. So, the goal should be to practice at least several times a week, even if only for short sessions.

3. Can yoga help with anxiety and depression? Some studies have proven that the usual practice of yoga counts a lot in decreasing stress and depression symptoms by helping a person relax and become more mindful and self-regulating.

4. Is it Safe to Practice with a Medical Condition? While generally

safe, always check with your healthcare provider before starting, especially with a pre-existing condition. A qualified teacher can help you tailor postures to your individual needs.

How am I supposed to quiet my mind during meditation if I cannot? Well, that will happen a lot in the beginning, but that's okay. When you notice your mind straying off, see it without judgment and gently bring your focus back to the breath. Over time, with practice, you'll find yourself more and more able to relax right into calm and clarity.

As the power of the vagus nerve-relaxation response reminder connection reminds us, our body is wise. In doing yoga, we tap into this wisdom as we find inner peace and enhance our resilience against the stresses of life. Thus, when you next find yourself in a stress whirlwind, pause, breathe deeply, and move mindfully to allow your vagus nerve to take you back to your natural calm state. Yoga and the Relaxation Response Herein lies the great need for yoga about the relaxation response and the vagus nerve—one from which we can draw on our body's wisdom and establish peaceful resilience against the sources of wear and tear. Next time you get tripped up in the storm of stress, remember: Stop. Breathe deep. Move with intention. and let your vagus nerve lead you back to that place of peace.

With time and patience, you can find an inner reservoir of peace you never knew you had.

An easy but very expressive yoga flow for spinal health, flexibility, and overall well-being is the Cat-Cow Pose. The benefits of Cat-Cow in daily practice are, from personal experience, the release of tension, improvement in posture, and deepening of the mind-body connection.

Cat-Cow, or Marjaryasana-Bitilasana in Sanskrit, describes a fundamental sequence of Hatha Yoga that exemplifies the innate quality of the cat—graceful, flexible, and adaptable in nature—as well as that of the cow—nourished, abundant, loving, and self-forgetting. It is through these qualities of the former to the latter that, as practitioners, we can cultivate balance, harmony, and resilience both on and off the mat in practice.

The benefits are manifold:

1. Maintaining the health and flexibility of the spine by lubricating the joints, promoting increased blood circulation, and stretching the muscles.

2. Improved posture due to easing tension, strengthening the core and aligning the upper body.

3. Relieves stress and induces relaxation through gentle, rhythmic movement, breath synchronization, and awareness of the present moment.

4. Improved emotional balance and heightened self-awareness are achieved by observing inner experiences with a detached curiosity.

5. To prepare the body and mind for deeper yoga practice.

Practice: Start in a quadruped position, with your knees under hips and hands under shoulders. Inhale as you tilt your tailbone and chest up towards the ceiling—create a curve in your back (Cow); exhale and round through the spine, tucking your chin and tailbone (Cat). Moving with your breath, transitioning from one shape to the next, noticing the sensations created within your spine as this happens, and encouraging a release of tension. Do this for 5–10 breaths or more, and then take a moment to relax in a neutral spine or Child's Pose.

Adapt as needed for your body:

- Reduction of pressure on wrists by padding or practicing on the forearms.

- Allow a soft gaze and support the head using props to relieve neck tension.

- Consider knee sensitivity in cushioning design or broader stance.

- Offer a seated variation on a chair or introduce some gentle twisting for variety.

Add Cat-Cow to your daily to-do list: wake up, break up your workday, wind down in the evening, or as a gentle transition between poses. Regular practice—even in small doses—has a powerful effect on overall well-being.

While yoga is suitable for most, when starting, especially if one has pre-existing conditions, consult with a qualified health provider and seek qualified teachers to tailor practices to your needs. Patience with the process—quite sometime later through practice—will be when the physical and mental benefits will start unfolding. This connection between the vagus nerve and the relaxation response reminds us that it's possible to tap into our bodies' deep state of ease and peace through mindful movement and breath. Keep practicing, let go, and the journey of Cat-Cow will bring you to a space inside that is more balanced, open-living, and resilient.

6.3 Child's Pose (Balasana)

In this quickly moving, high-stress world, we lose touch with our calm center. We tend to jump from one commitment to the other, pushing or instead punishing ourselves to the extreme, more often than not, in neglect of the whisper of our body and mind. But it also contains a simple, straightforward button to press, one that allows access to our innate ability to be at peace and to be free from inner turmoil: Child's Pose, or Balasana in Sanskrit, a deeply restorative, nourishing practice, one that soothes frayed nerves, tensions, and cultivates an innermost sense of peacefulness.

As one whom herself has often experienced the transforming power of Child's Pose, I can attest to its remarkable ability to soothe the nervous system, quiet the mind, and yoke the body-mind into a deep state of rest and renewal. We will discuss its many benefits, its simple and potent capability, step-by-step instructions on performing this posture, and how it gets integrated into our self-care toolkit.

Balasana is a simple asana under Hatha yoga. Balasana gets its name from the Sanskrit words "Bala," which means child, and "asana," which means posture.

The pose mimics a child in the fetal position in the womb: knees bent, pulled in under the belly; the forehead rests on the ground with arms just by the side of the body. This introspective, almost fetal position would be considered safe, with a surrendering feeling of nurturing and safety, touching into our inner child in its innocence.

Child's Pose is a representation of letting go. We fold inward and place the forehead on the earth, creating humility, vulnerability, and deep self-acceptance in understanding that we don't have to always be in charge—we can take a break, buoyed by the supportive ground under us.

Though it may be a simple pose, Child's Pose can work wonders:

1. Calm and Soothe the Nervous System: To its very nature and function, the pose calls forth the action of the parasympathetic nervous system—to arise—in the "rest and digest" state. By slowing one's breathing, releasing tension in the body, and promoting safety and grounding, Child's Pose shifts us into a state of relaxation and recovery, which is crucial in today's world of chronic stress.

2. Releases Tension Across the Body: It provides a slight stretch across the back, hips, thighs, and ankles while releasing tension across the neck and shoulders. The weight of the forehead may also release tension from the brow and jaw.

3. Inducing Introspection and Self-Reflexivity: By turning inwards and giving in to being held by the earth, space is created to delve into our inner landscape—thoughts, feelings, and sensations. This self-inquiry becomes a way to cultivate insight into emotional patterns and triggers, resulting in clarity, compassion, and resilience.

4. Improving Sleep and Relaxation: If done before bed, Child's Pose relaxes the mind and releases tension, enabling the body to sleep more soundly. The gentle pressure on the forehead works on the pineal gland by increasing the secretory action, which helps in the sleep-wake cycle. The feelings of grounding and safety created in this posture are particularly soothing for insomnia or nighttime anxiety.

To Do Child's Pose:

1. Kneel with the big toes touching, the knees hip-width apart. A blanket or cushion can be used under the knees for padding.

2. Exhale, lowering torso forward, resting forehead on the floor or block/blanket/cushion for support. Arms will be relaxed alongside the body, with the palms facing up and the fingers soft.

3. Get comfortable in the pose. Feel how your weight drops to the ground. Sensation spots tension and consciously asks it to let go with every exhale.

4. Practice slow, deep, gentle breathing. Allow the breath to fill the back body on the inhale and the belly to draw back toward the spine on the exhale gently. Use the breath as an anchor, smoothly leading the way to relaxation.

5. Breathe and hold for 5 to 10 breaths or longer. To release, press your hands into the ground and lift your torso to a kneeling position, pausing to notice sensations of openness, release, or calm.

Adapt the pose to your needs.

- Wide-Legged: Take with wider knees, letting your belly come in between your thighs. This will be helpful for those who have tight hips, lower backs, large bodies, or pregnancy.

- Supported: put block under forehead, chest or hips, cushion, blanket for support and accessibility.

- Arms Overhead: Reach arms forward to increase stretch on shoulder/upper back area.

- Fists Under Forehead: Place fists them under the forehead for support and cushioning, particularly when one has forehead or neck discomfort.

The key here is to find a variation that feels safe, comfortable, and nourishing for your unique body and needs. Experiment with modifications until you find what works best.

Add Child's Pose to your daily practice.

- As a morning wake-up, gently bringing sleep into awake-ness while providing a sense of peace and grounding for the day.

- During work breaks – releasing tension, refreshing energy, refocusing the mind.

- In the evening wind-down routine, releasing stresses of the day, calming the nervous system, and preparing for restful sleep.

- Transition pose, pausing, breathing, reconnecting, moving with intention and awareness.

Remember: practice being consistent. Well-being and overall health—just a couple of minutes a day in Child's pose can have a tremendous effect over a lifetime.

Child's Pose is generally safe for most and is accessible to most people, but approach with caution if you have injuries or sensitivities to the knees, neck, or back. Use props to come out of the pose if you feel sharp pain or discomfort in your body. Use caution if you have previous conditions and ideally seek guidance from a health professional or a qualified yoga teacher. Adjust the position of the knees as necessary for pregnancy. Other adaptations to experiment with are using props under the hips. Again, always refer to your providers. If you don't feel relaxed in the pose, remember to approach the experience with curiosity and self-compassion, to feel and acknowledge whatever arises without trying to change it. A fantastic way to focus and still the mind and body in the present moment is to focus on breath or a calming affirmation. Be reminded that yoga is not the cultivation of some state but of awareness, acceptance, and compassion for who we are.

One may generally think that Child's Pose is such an easy asana, but the power it holds toward transforming physical, mental, and emotional well-being is not one to underestimate. By surrendering to the moment and letting go of tension and resistance, we tap into deep wells of our inner peace, resilience, and self-nurturing that can ripple into every other aspect of our lives.

So the next time you feel overwhelmed, anxious, or disconnected, take a few moments in Child's Pose. Root down, let go of everything, and simply be held by the loving embrace of the supporting ground. Exhale and feel the body and mind release and open even more, making way for an abundance of ease, clarity, and joy.

6.4 Standing Forward Bend (Uttanasana)

It's as if you were a tree: your body rooted deeply in the ground, arms extended to the sky, moved by the breeze, bent and fluid with every blow. This is the essence of the posture Uttanasana, also known as Standing Forward Bend: rooted in an invitation to let go and surrender into NOW.

Having experienced the power of Uttanasana myself, I can clearly say that it is intense in calming the mind, releasing bodily tension, and enhancing activity in the vagus nerve—a significant component of the parasympathetic nervous system, stimulating the "rest and digest" response. In this fingerstand, we will cover the myriad benefits of what appears to be such a simple pose, detailed step-by-step instructions for its safe and effective practice, and how it can become an essential tool for self-care and the regulation of the nervous system.

Uttanasana is one of the standing asanas in Hatha Yoga. Hatha Yoga is an all-embracing practice based on asana (physical pose), pranayama (breath work), and a calm, clear mind. The word "Uttanasana" is derived from Sanskrit words: "ut" means intense, "tan" means to stretch or extend, and "asana" means posture.

The shape is a deep forward fold, with the upper body folding over legs and hands reaching toward the feet or floor. This can be a very intense hamstring, calf, and lower back stretch, but it is also very powerful.

On a deeper level, Uttanasana is a letting-go posture. We forward bend, bowing to the wisdom of the body and the present moment, like this liberating us from the clutches of ego and the illusion of control. It can be very transformative, helping us to develop humility, trust, and acceptance about the multiplicity and diversity of difficulties and uncertainties life brings.

uttanasana gives numerous benefits:

1. Soothing the Nervous System: Bending forward and gently compressing the abdominal organs stimulates the vagal response; the signal travels to the brain, which starts the "rest and digest" parasympathetic system. The tilt in the dominance toward the parasympathetic system decreases cortisol, cools inflammation, and turns on overall calming and well-being in both mind and body, making it vital in the modern world of stress and anxiety.

Stretch out and lengthen the body: The intense stretch of this pose for the legs, back, and neck improves flexibility, reduces muscle tension and stiffness, and helps prevent injury. It is very useful for individuals who are in a sitting or standing position for long periods to counter poor posture and alignment.

3. Improvement of digestion and elimination: the delicate compression in the abdomen stimulates the digestive system, encourages peristalsis or wave-like contraction of food through the intestines, releasing tension and stagnation in the gut, improving circulation, and promoting a sense of lightness and ease in the body, helpful for digestive issues like bloating, constipation, or IBS.

4 Reducing stress and anxiety: The posture activates the parasympathetic nervous system, inducing a grounded, stable, and calm state to use against the stress response, quieting the mind, reducing agitation and overwhelm, promoting inner peace and resilience in the face of life's challenges. The calming forward fold helps to bring both mind and emotions inwards,

supporting introspection and self-reflection, something constructive during times of uncertainty or transition when we may feel unmoored or disconnected from our inner knowing.

5. Reduces Headaches and Fatigue: The pose sends more blood to your head and face, thus relieving tension headaches. It seems that one's clarity and focus are recharged. The gentle inversion reduces feelings of fatigue, enlivens the body, encourages fresh blood flow to the brain, and promotes oxygen to be absorbed into tissues in the body. This is especially good during stress or overwork when we feel depleted or burned out.

To do Uttanasana:

Begin in Tadasana (Mountain Pose), with your feet hip-distance apart and hands by your sides—the sensation of rooting down through your feet and lengthening up through.

2. Inhale, stretch your arms out and up over the head, reaching toward the sky.

3. Exhale, hinging at hips, with long spin and engaged core; arms fall forward and reach the ground.

4. Bend the knees as much as needed to take the fold over the legs: the back should stay straight, and the neck should hang. Press the hands into the shins, ankles, or blocks to take some of them.

5. Let head hang heavy, feelings of tension in the neck and shoulders release. If you need to, sway or nod your head gently to let go of any tightness.

6. Exhale, letting the body sink into the stretch. Every inhale lengthens the spine and opens the chest. Every exhale, release, and surrender a little deeper into the fold.

7. To come out, hands on the waist, slowly vertebra by vertebra coming up, feeling the rooted feet and the tall spine before the arms release down to the sides.

Modify Uttanasana to suit you:

- Knees: May want to be bent if hamstrings or lower back are too tight or painful. Bend the knees quite a bit so the upper body can fold down relatively comfortably and slowly straighten them out again as the flexibility gets better.

Use a block: If the floor is too far away for the hands, use a block or a pile of books to support the hands, allowing a reach with less strain toward the lower back and a deep stretch through the hamstrings and calves.

- Widen your stance. Your inner thighs feel tight, and/or it is just a struggle to point the hips toward your body. So, widen the stance slightly more than hip distanced to get more significant space in the pelvis and achieve a better inner thigh stretch.

- Fold arms: If there is any shoulder or wrist pain, fold the arms behind the back, clasping opposite elbows. That will release the tension from the upper body and let the stretching focus on the legs and lower back.

- Twist: Allow for a twist by reaching the right hand toward the left ankle or shin and the left hand toward the right ankle or shin so that the torso is allowed to twist gently from side to side; it is a deep spinal stretch and a gentle massage for the organs.

Do not sacrifice your comfort or safety for some idea of the outward form of the pose.

Make Uttanasana part of your daily routine:

• As a morning wake-up to bring the body to life, stimulate digestion, and set a grounded, centered tone for the day.

• At midday, as a tension-releasing reset, energy-refreshing reset, and mind-refocusing reset.

• As an evening wind-down, let the stressors of the day fall away. Calm the nervous system in preparation for restorative sleep.

• Between activities or postures — as a transition and to pause, to bring the mind back to the breath, to set intentionality, and to move with awareness.

Being consistent is the key: A few minutes of Uttanasana daily will profoundly impact general, physical, mental, and emotional well-being over time.

While generally safe for most, approach with caution if you have any eye condition such as glaucoma or detached retina, or serious neck injuries. In case of pre-existing health concerns, get in touch with your healthcare provider or a qualified yoga instructor before the commencement of the pose. Adapt as necessary in pregnancy, adding a bolster or blankets under the hips with a gentle slope to the floor rather than having the legs entirely against the wall. Always listen to your body and consult with your providers before starting any new practice.

Although it appears to be just a simple forward bend, the power of uttanasana to transform physical, mental, and emotional well-being is not to be underestimated. With this surrender to gravity, release of tension and resistance, and stimulation of the vagus nerve, we stumble upon a great well of inner peace, resilience, and vitality.

So, the next time you feel all tensed up, anxious, and disconnected from body and breath, simply practice Uttanasana right then and there. Just let yourself root down. Let go of any tension or holding in the body that doesn't serve this moment of being; just let it go. Let your body and mind release and open with every breath out, allowing more room to accommodate ease, clarity, and joy.

Remember that your practice is an exploration of self-discovery and acceptance. There is no perfect Uttanasana; there is no final destination—just meet yourself with curiosity, compassion, and an open heart, trusting that your practice will meet you exactly where you are.

May this Uttanasana nourish and heal you, be ground for transformation, and invoke a deeper relationship with yourself, your body, your breath, and the world around you. With practice and patience, you may realize that inverting one's perspective on and off the mat would mean problems are but only opportunities for growth and not setbacks, and from rest, one must be nourished. And, remember always, you are whole, worthy, and enough just as you are.

So allow yourself to rest, relax, and just be. Go along with Uttanasana toward your self-discovery and self-care. Trust that with every breath, with every pause, you're sowing the seeds for a much greater life of peace, resilience, and joy.

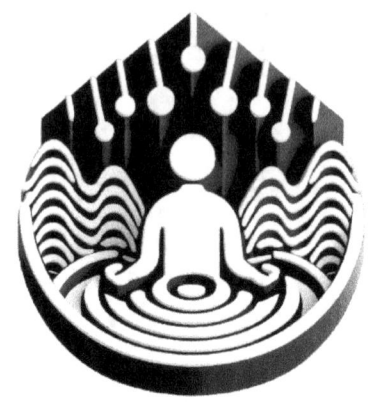

Chapter 7

Sound Therapy and Chanting or Vagus Nerve Stimulation

Welcome to the incredible journey of the deep connection between sound, the vagus nerve, and your whole-well-being.

At the heart of it, though, is the vagus nerve—one of the most prominent nerves of our autonomic nervous system. This long, wandering nerve that meanders from the brainstem to all over the body—innervating specific target organs—plays a vital role in controlling heart rate, digestion, and immunity. A well-toned, properly working vagus nerve will bring a person into a state of relaxation, reduce inflammation, and create a healthier being.

Research confirms how specific frequencies and tones can elicit the vagus nerve to its soothing, restorative effect on the body. For example, it has been found that listening to low-frequency sounds produced by singing bowls or chanting increases heart rate variability, a marker of healthy vagal tone. A higher HRV is related to more stress resilience better emotional regulation, and higher well-being.

However the benefits of sound therapy go far beyond relaxation. Studies have also shown that it can help reduce symptoms associated with anxiety, depression, and post-traumatic stress disorder (PTSD). Another fascinating area of research into the impact of sound is on the brain itself. Using advanced imaging techniques, such as functional MRI (fMRI), scientists have found that listening to music or tones can activate specific brain regions linked to emotion, memory, and reward.

This is important because the vagus nerve can only be triggered or activated by some sounds. While some frequencies and certain tones are proven therapeutic, others have little or no effect and may even have a counterproductive effect. This is where a trained, sound therapist can be worth their weight in gold: customizing the experience to your personal needs and goals.

In addition to working with sound therapists, there are numerous ways to bring sound therapy into your daily life. In a schedule packed with very little time, it sometimes only takes a few minutes of listening to calming music or sounds of nature to impact your stress and overall sense of well-being significantly. You might even consider using singing bowls, tuning forks, or simply your voice in creating experiences with vibrational healing.

As with any new practice, it is always best to take it slowly at first and to heed the messages of your own body. It couldn't hurt to chat with your healthcare provider before taking up any new therapy in case you have preexisting health conditions or other worries.

The science behind sound therapy and its effect on the vagus nerve allows for it to make a compelling statement regarding sound's healing and transformative ability. Sound can be used to activate the vagus nerve, triggering the relaxation response, and may be used in the support of general health and well-being. Whether you are looking for remedies against stress and anxiety or chronic pains, or you just want to improve your quality of life, sound therapy might be a gentle and effective way out.

Let's continue to explore the world of sound healing: feel welcome to be curious, open, and compassionate with yourself. Remember that healing is a journey, not a destination and that every small step toward greater well-being is a cause for celebration.

May the power of sound guide you as you journey through the experiences awaiting your perfect health, joy, and spirit.

7.1 Humming and Its Effects on Vagal Tone

Let's go to the basics. Humming produces a continuous sound with your voice by closing the lips and allowing the vocal cords to vibrate. This is a natural, easy way to vocalize, something that has been practiced for centuries across many different cultures, including music and healing practices.

But really, what goes on in your body that causes you to hum? When you hum, the vocal cords are vibrating, which produces a gentle vibration in the entire body. It is most strongly experienced in the chest, throat, and face from the vibration.

Physiologically, humming involves some significant muscles and structures making voice. In other words, humming engages the diaphragm: the big muscle at the bottom of the lungs, which contracts and relaxes as one breathes in and out. This deep, rhythmic breathing stimulates the vagus nerve, which runs from the brainstem to the abdomen and is vital in controlling the autonomic nervous system.

Call it the body's internal 'chill-out' button. A vagus nerve, when triggered, is said to slow the heart, reduce blood pressure, and instill a sense of well-being by generating relaxation. This is where the magic of humming comes in. It is even hypothesized that vibrations caused by humming might stimulate the vagus nerve and increase its tone, thus restoring calm and a sense of well-being.

The benefits of humming do not stop here. Humming is also capable of:

• Alleviating stress and anxiety

•Improve quality of

• Improve the immune system

•Enhance oxygenation and circulation

• Mental clarity and concentration

- Relieve pain and tension

So, how are you going to implement humming in your everyday life to realize these incredible gains? The great news is, it's straightforward :.

Here is a simple humming exercise that you can try right away:

Step or lie down in a silent, comfortable place.

2. With a deep breath, close your eyes as you breathe fully into your lungs, allowing your body to feel still and relaxed.

3. Close your mouth slowly and hum comfortably and enjoyably resonant.

4. Concentrate on the body's vibrations, particularly in the region of the chest and the throat.

5.Keep humming for 5-10 minutes, depending on how long you feel comfortable with.

6. When you are ready to finish, take a few deep breaths and gently open your eyes, noticing how your body feels.

You can do this simple humming exercise anywhere and anytime: when sitting at one's desk at work, resting on a busy day, or even before going to sleep. Do whatever it takes to make this one more regular thing in your self-care toolbox.

Now, I know what some of you might be thinking. "But Tom, I can't carry a tune to save my life! Will I not sound ridiculous while humming?" The thing is, it doesn't matter how you sound in humming. You are not trying to win a Grammy here. The beauty of it is that you create some kind of vibration within your body to harvest its therapeutic benefits.

It has been shown that humming, even at a low frequency of around 130 Hz, can still help activate the vagus nerve to effect relaxation. Such a frequency is well within the range of what most people would hum naturally.

Another common concern is whether humming can be done discretely enough that nobody would notice. You most definitely can. You can hum quietly enough that only you can hear it, making it an excellent tool for stress relief in public places like the office or public transportation.

Any time you feel self-conscious about how you are humming, remember that this is an entirely natural and innate human activity. The majority of infants frequently hum as part of their self-pleasuring activities, and many ethnic groups throughout the world use humming as an integral part of their music and healing traditions.

So do give it a try. Start with humming for a few minutes a day and then slowly increase the duration of your humming time over several days if necessary to make it comfortable for you. Be mindful of what occurs in your body, and remember which changes you note in your mood, energy level, or general state of being.

7.2 Chanting "OM" for Vagus Nerve Stimulation

Have you ever felt a deep sense of serenity wash over you after chanting "OM"? That's not by any coincidence. The vibrations through this ancient sound stimulate your vagus nerve, which helps regulate your autonomic nervous system into relaxed states. In this section, we will trace the history of the "OM" chant, learn the correct way to sing it and see how it can be implemented as a tool to assist in gaining an improvement in your all-over state of well-being.

The Meaning and Origins of "OM"

The sound "OM" (also written as "AUM") has a rich history dating back thousands of years. It is considered one of the most sacred sounds in various spiritual traditions, including Hinduism, Buddhism, and Jainism. The syllable "OM" is believed to represent the primordial sound of the universe, encompassing all of creation.

Each letter of "OM" holds a specific meaning:

- "A" represents the waking state, the physical realm.
- "U" represents the dream state, the mental realm.
- "M" represents the deep sleep state, the spiritual realm.

When these three sounds are combined, they symbolize the totality of existence and the unity of all things. Chanting "OM" is thought to connect us with this universal energy, promoting feelings of peace, harmony, and oneness.

The Science Behind "OM" Chanting

Some recent scientific studies are beginning to reveal these physiological effects of chanting "OM." One recently published in the International

Journal of Yoga indicated the "potential benefits" of chanting "OM" regularly, which includes effects like reducing stress, anxiety, and depression while improving overall well-being.

In another study, researchers from the University of California at San Diego discovered that "OM" could trigger activity in the vagus nerve, thereby increasing heart rate variability (HRV) and enhancing autonomic regulation. HRV is the variation in time between heartbeats, where higher HRV is associated with better health and stress resilience.

There is generally a belief among many that these vibrations set by chanting the sound "OM" excite the vagus nerve due to a phenomenon known as "binaural synchronization." The sound vibrations of "OM" pass through the vocal cords, sinuses, and skull, causing subtle vibrations in the ear canal. Then, this vibration frequency is caught up by the vagus nerve, which in turn signals the brain to calm down into a parasympathetic state gradually.

How to Chant OM for Vagus Nerve Stimulation

Now that we have understood the science behind "OM" chanting, we shall go through the proper technique for vagus nerve stimulation by "OM" chanting. Here's a simple step-by-step procedure:

1. Find a quiet, comfortable space, free from distraction, in which you can sit cross-legged on the floor, on a cushion, or in a chair—both feet flat on the ground.

2. Close your eyes and breathe deeply, allowing your body to settle and release into relaxation.

3.Inhale deeply through your nostrils with your mouth closed so that you fill your lungs with air.

4.Breathe very slowly and chant "OM" as long as possible. It should resonate deep in your belly, chest, and throat.

5.Let the sound fade with its own volition toward the last part of your exhalation.

6. Do another deep breath, and repeat the chant, tuning into the vibrations and sensations in your ENTIRE body.

7.Then continue with the chanting "OM" throughout for 5-10 minutes, perhaps even longer for you.

8.And when you're ready to finish, take a few deep breaths and gently open your eyes, allowing yourself a moment to observe any changes there might be in your physical, mental, or emotional state.

Tips to Improve Your OM ChANT

• Play with pitch and volume to locate the resonance that feels best and most empowering.

• Group chanting of "OM" has been considered very effective since the collective energy increases the magnitude of positive vibrations.

• Include the chanting of "OM" in a more exciting way by including other kinds of activities that stimulate the vagus nerve, such as deep breathing or even gentle neck stretches.

• Let the chanting of "OM" be a routine, even for some minutes, every day.

7.3 Singing Bowls and Their Influence on the Autonomic Nervous System

Imagine this: you're sitting with your eyes closed in a silent room, a singing bowl emitting a gentle sound wave. The harmonious waves have already filled the room; you are beginning to feel your body relaxing, your mind calming down, and a sense of complete peace falling into the bones. My friends, this is the magic with singing bowls, ancient instruments that have the profound capacity to influence our autonomic nervous system toward relaxation.

The Origins of Singing Bowls

Singing bowls, also called Tibetan or Himalayan bowls, have a relatively long and rich history in terms of centuries and across different cultures. Although the exact origins of these instruments are somewhat mysterious, some say that they first emerged in the Himalayan regions of Tibet, Nepal, and India as early as the 10th century BC.

Singing bowls were traditionally made from a mixture of various metals: copper, tin, zinc, iron, and sometimes with the addition of gold or silver. They were used in antiquity for meditation and spiritual healing. It is because of this mixture of materials, the ratio in this mixture, the thickness of the metals, and the size that singing bowls get their unique acoustic properties, producing a rich and complex sound full of overtones.

Traditionally, in Buddhist circles, singing bowls were a focal point for many mindfulness and meditation practices. Striking or circling the bowl's rim with a mallet smoothes the mind, develops a sense of presence, and promotes feelings of deep inner peace. They would ring at the beginning and end of periods of silent contemplation, chanting, and other spiritual exercises.

Apart from the religious context, the bowls had healing qualities. According to Tibetan medicine, the vibrations made by the bowls would harmonize all the body's energy centers and give rise to physical, emotional, and spiritual benefits. A practitioner would thus place the bowl upon the body directly or even close to the body so that resonant frequencies would penetrate it, bringing back into line the natural rhythms in the body.

The Science of Sound and the Autonomic Nervous System

Western science has merely started to catch up to insights that have long been an integral part of ancient wisdom traditions: that sound has a profound impact on our physiology and mental states. At the heart of this connection lies the autonomic nervous system.

The autonomic nervous system regulates most of the unconscious but critical processes the body performs: heart rate, digestion, and respiration. It has two departments: The sympathetic nervous system operates in stress-borne circumstances and prepares for action, while the parasympathetic one carries out relaxation and restoration.

It is in those moments that we are under chronic stress and anxiety that our sympathetic nervous system tends to go on overdrive. We feel this in several physical and emotional symptoms: tension, fatigue, irritability, and sleeplessness. This is the power of singing bowls.

Research has shown that the vibrations caused by the singing bowls can directly influence the autonomic nervous system, bringing the body out of the state of sympathetic dominance into the state of parasympathetic ease. A published study in the Journal of Evidence-Based Complementary & Alternative Medicine pointed out that subjects undergoing a singing bowl sound meditation exhibited a significant increase in heart rate variability—one of the critical markers of parasympathetic activity and resilience to stress.

But how do singing bowls affect the nervous system? This is due to the acoustic features of the instruments and their ability to stimulate the vagus nerve.

This is the most prolonged and most complex of all the cranial nerves. It extends from the brainstem to the neck, chest, and abdomen, being involved with and contributing to the functioning of many systems that support life in the body: heart rate, digestion, and so on. When the vagus nerve is activated, it coaxes the brain into relaxation, dampening stress levels and keeping the person's cheerfulness up.

One of the critical ways that singing bowls stimulate the vagus nerve is through the phenomenon of "entrainment." Entrainment is the body's tendency to sync with the external rhythmic stimulus about physiological rhythms, including brain waves and heartbeat. This explanation is consistent with how listening to the soft tones from a singing bowl quiets the mind, gets the brainwaves to slow down to match the frequency of the sound, and essentially leads individuals into a very relaxed and peaceful inner state.

DO Singing Bowls into Your Practice

Now that we've learned the science behind singing bowls and how these affect the autonomic nervous system, let's look at some practical ways to use these tools for your wellness practice.

1. Choose the suitable bowl: Singing bowls come in different sizes, shapes, and materials, and all these features give a unique character and specific acoustic properties to any bowl. When buying one, follow your inner voice and select the one you feel most gently. Take the bowl gently into your hands and tap it with a mallet lightly, noticing the sound you are receiving from it. A high-quality bowl should produce a clear, prolonged sound, which is lovely and smooth to your ears, and make it while feeling the vibrations in your body.

Create a Sacred Space: For the highest experience from your practice, set an atmosphere that is undisturbed and profoundly nourishing, allowing yourself to relax and let go. Find a nice, quiet spot in your home and make the environment more welcoming with soft lighting, cozy cushions, and your favorite aromatherapy scents. The more your space feels welcoming and nutritious, the more quickly you will slip into a deep state of relaxation.

3. Set an intention: Just before you start your singing bowl meditation, make a reconnection to your breath and set an intention—clearly, for your practice. You can do this simply by stating, "I'm open to my peace and healing," or "I release all physical and emotional tension from my body and mind." This way, you'll have something pointed to guide you along during your session, keeping you aligned and present.

4. Strike the bowl and listen deeply: There are so many ways to play a singing bowl, but one of the simplest, most effective ways is to strike the rim of the bowl softly with a mallet and then let the sound come alive and fade away on its own. Feel how your body responds to those soothing tones, even how your breath changes, how the energy in the air changes. And if your mind begins to wander, bring it back to the bowl's sound.

5. Experiment with placement: You can also hold the bowl right on your body or over an area that is tense or blocked. For instance, on your chest if you're trying to breathe deeply and relax; on your belly, if things are rough digestion-wise. Follow your intuition and allow your body to guide you to the placement that feels most nourishing and supportive.

6. Combine with other practices: Singing bowls are good partners with other mindfulness and self-care practices, like meditation, yoga, or qi gong. Try adding the calming tones of the bowl into your daily routine, and notice how this can enrich your essential well-being and vitality.

So look further into the world of the singing bowl and sound healing knowing that the most important thing is to approach your practice with an open heart and spirit of curiosity. There is no right or wrong way—it's very sacred. Only trust your inner wisdom and be guided by what supports you most and feels most nourishing.

With time and practice, you might find that the gentle vibrations of the singing bowl become a friend, dearer to you on your healing and self-discovery journey, bringing you to a place of peace, presence, and harmony deep within.

So go ahead, strike that bowl, close your eyes, and let the magic of sound wash over you.

7.4 Tuning Forks for Vagus Nerve Activation

In sound therapy, tuning forks have become a potent tool for engendering a relaxed and balanced state in which general well-being can be restored. These superficial yet profound instruments have been used for centuries for the tuning of musical instruments, but their healing application has been, until recently, virtually undiscovered.

Sound therapy with tuning forks mainly acts based on the principle of resonance: all objects have a particular natural frequency at which they vibrate—just like the human body. We use very exact frequencies emitted by tuning forks to help our body return to balance and harmony for health and well-being on a physical, mental, and emotional level.

A fantastic application for the tuning fork developed in the last years is in stimulations towards the vagus nerve, the central nerve of the organism during the regulation of the body's stress response in the parasympathetic nervous system. We've learned in other places that the vagus nerve drives the system in regulating the body's stress response in an organism. That means that toning the vagus nerve can have profound effects on our health and well-being.

So, how do tuning forks work in stimulating the vagus nerve? Let's probe into the principles and applications of this exciting therapy.

The Science of Sound and Vibration

Understanding how tuning forks can affect the vagus nerve involves looking at the science of sound and vibration first. A sound is thus a form in which a vibration travels through a medium—a gas, liquid, or solid. Waves, when they propagate, carry a design of hertz, which will be their frequency and, therefore, determine their pitch.

Every object, including our bodies, has a natural frequency at which it vibrates. That entrainment effect occurs when we subject our bodies to an external frequency that matches or harmonizes with our natural frequency. Our body simply starts to vibrate in tune with the external frequency, a process that brings balance, relaxation, and restoration to the body.

Tuning forks are designed to produce pure, exact frequency to focus and entrain areas of the body. When struck and placed on or near the body, these tuning forks introduce a gentle vibration experienced on the skin and further into the tissues and organs.

Vagus Nerve and Sound Therapy

New research has demonstrated an exciting influence pattern on the vagus nerve within specific frequencies, namely the low range below 100 Hz. Stimulation of the vagus nerve induces the parasympathetic nervous system, which takes on the body's functions in the state of "rest and digest" to get active.

Under parasympathetic dominance, the body is in a state that is conducive to experiencing the following benefits therapeutically:

• Decreased heart rate and blood pressure

• Enhanced blood flow to the digestive organs

- Reduced inflammation

- Increased immune function

- Feelings of increased calm and relaxation

The use of tuning fork stimulations for the vagus nerve can be done to support the state of parasympathetic tone and the numerous benefits it brings.

Using tuning forks for vagal nerve stimulation

Here are a few simple techniques:

1. Behind the ear: The vagus nerve runs behind the ear and down the neck. Strike a low-frequency tuning fork (128 Hz or 64 Hz) and gently place it behind your ear. Hold it there for 30-60 seconds or until the vibration dissipates.

In the chest: And the vagus also connects to your heart and lungs. Try putting a low-frequency tuning fork on your chest and holding it for several deep breaths.

3. On the abdomen: The vagus nerve provides innervation to the enteric plexus, the modulator of digestion and gut motility. Hold a low-pitched tuning fork over your abdomen at the level of the umbilicus and take deep, slow breaths into your abdomen.

4. Spine: The vagus nerve is located running down both sides of the spine. Stimulation can help to relax the body. Start a low-frequency tuning fork

at the base of the spine and travel slowly up the spine, pausing for several seconds at each vertebra.

Of course, like any new therapy, it is essential to start slowly and listen to what your body is telling you. For any pre-existing conditions that you may have or any doubts about using tuning fork therapy, professional healthcare guidance is always advisable.

7.5 Binaural Beats and Vagal Tone

Have you ever considered an influence exerted on your mind and body that could be effected through sound alone? Enter binaural beats: a curious auditory phenomenon that has gained popularity in past years for its potential to increase relaxation, focus, and even vagal tone. In this section, we get under the skin of the science behind binaural beats, learn how you can use them to foster autonomic regulation and get practical tips on how to integrate them into your life.

What Exactly are Binaural Beats

Binaural beats are a kind of auditory illusion coming from two separately played, slightly different frequencies into each ear. For example, if a 200 Hz frequency is played in the left ear and a 210 Hz frequency is played in the right ear, the brain is going to perceive what the illusory third beat frequency of 10 Hz is; these frequencies are the difference between the two initial frequencies.

An auditory beat frequency is set up, not in the physical vibratory sounds outside the body but within the brain. The theory behind binaural beats is quite simple: if you listen to some frequency, somehow the brain entrains its brainwaves to that same frequency, and mental and physiological states are somehow altered.

Binaural beat frequencies can be classified into four key categories, which consciousness states can be described as:

1. Delta waves (0.5-4 Hz): Associated with deep sleep, relaxation, and healing.

2. Theta waves (4-8 Hz): Associated with deep meditation, creativity, and emotional connection.

3. Alpha waves (8-13 Hz): Associated with relaxation, stress reduction, and learning.

4. Beta waves (13-30 Hz): Associated with alertness, concentration, and problem-solving.

By listening to binaural beats in these different frequency ranges, we can potentially influence our brainwave patterns and promote specific states of mind and body.

The Vagus Nerve Connection

Some recent studies have also shown that by listening to some binaural beats with the same frequency on both ears, this vagus nerve stimulation can be influenced, and the vagal tone is increased.

A published study in Frontiers in Neuroscience has revealed that binaural beats in the alpha frequency range (10 Hz) increased heart rate variability (HRV) significantly while reducing self-reported anxiety in subjects. This would suggest that HRV is the prime marker of vagal tone and autonomic regulation in that higher levels of HRV equal a better ability to cope with stress and, overall, good health.

In another study, University of Otago New Zealand researchers found that listening to binaural beats in the theta frequency (7 Hz) was associated with increased parasympathetic activity and decreased sympathetic activity in participants. The vagus nerve mediates the parasympathetic nervous system and provides relaxation and recovery, while the sympathetic nervous system deals with the stress response of "fight or flight.".

Taken together, these results support the notion that specific frequencies of binaural beats could be eliciting a response in the Vagus Nerve—subsequently improving HRV and general states of relaxation/stress resilience.

How to Use Binaural Beats for Vagal Tone

The binaural beats are most effective, and their full effects are realized only, when one is using stereo headphones. In this way, the different frequencies are played separately into your ears, creating the desired beat frequency in the brain.

Choose from the varieties of binaural beat recordings available online once you have your headphones or through mobile applications. Here's how you make your choice on binaural beats and how you use them:

1.Choose a frequency range depending on what state you would like to be in, either of your mind or body. For vagal tone and relaxation, alpha or theta frequencies are an excellent place to start.

2. Get into a quiet, relaxed position, sitting or lying down, where you will not be disturbed.

3 Begin with a very short listening period, 5-10 minutes; you can gradually lengthen the time by a sentence or two when you feel ready. Some people like 20-30 minutes in duration.

4. Combine binaural beats with relaxation methods, such as deep breathing and gentle stretching.

5. Patience and Consistency: Any new practice takes time to show results. One must listen to binaural beats regularly, for a few minutes every day.

Vagal Tone and Binaural Beats: Do They Make an Auditory Dream Team?

As we have detailed in this chapter, binaural beats provide an exciting and potentially potent means of entraining the brain to influence our mental and physiological states. This way, we can tap into different states of consciousness, from relaxation to focusing on the vagal tone of our brain, by entraining our brainwaves to particular frequencies.

The most exciting emerging research will associate a potential link between binaural beats and the vagus nerve, a straightforward and highly accessible way of supporting autonomic regulation and resilience to stress. With binaural beats, we incorporate them into our everyday lives, and we can develop a much greater sense of calm and balance.

A tool as new and strange as binaural beats needs treatment with an open mind and much self-experimentation. What works for one person may not work for another, and it might take a lot of trial and error to find the frequencies and durations of listening that work best with his needs and preferences.

So, why not give binaural beats a shot and observe their effect on you, your state of mind, and your body? Whether it is reducing stress, increasing your focus, or enhancing vagal tone, these entrancing auditory illusions might be the answer to unlocking your full potential.

Treat the practice with patience, curiosity, and self-compassion. Do trust that your body and mind know precisely what they need and that by tapping into the power of sound, you're taking an active role in your health and happiness.

Enjoy listening!

7.6 Gregorian Chants and Their Impact on the Parasympathetic Nervous System

In a fast-changing world like today, we often feel cut off and unrooted from ancient times. Or what if I told you that one of the world's oldest musical traditions could help you face the stresses common today and give you more balance and resilience in life? Enter the Gregorian chants: this form of religious music is both hauntingly beautiful and has accompanied the layman through the centuries by being instrumental, even if unwittingly, in providing him with relaxation, spiritual connection, and, yes, even vagus nerve-stimulating effects. To follow, the origin and nature of the Gregorian chant shall be revealed, supported by scientific facts as to how it affects the parasympathetic nervous system and suggestions on how to apply these enchanting melodies in everyday life.

The Timeless Beauty of Gregorian Chants

Gregorian chants are monophonic, unaccompanied sacred music originating from the Roman Catholic Church that existed in the 9th and 10th centuries. So named after the pope, Gregory I, who was popularly known to have collected and codified these chants, they were initially and traditionally performed in monasteries and churches across Europe by male monks singing in Latin.

The most distinctive feature of Gregorian chants is arguably the scale used to create another strange, otherworldly sound that's both haunting and profoundly relaxing. Unlike modern Western music, which is divided into primary or minor scales, Gregorian chants are composed in eight modes, each with a distinctive emotional flavor and melodic form.

One of the critical features of Gregorian chants involves the long melismas, where, in the course of the text, few lines are featured on more than one note per syllable. This creates a flowing, almost hypnotic effect that can help to quiet the mind and promote a state of deep relaxation.

Yet, more than anything else, Gregorian chants are not just beautiful to the ears; they have been tested and proved to have an absolute physiological impact on the body, especially regarding the parasympathetic nervous system and stimulating the vagus nerve.

Sounds and the Vagus Nerve: The Science

New studies have started to recognize sound's profound effects on our autonomic nervous system. One of them is the vagus nerve—the long, wandering nerve that is the primary conduit between the brain and the body's inner landscape.

In one study published in the Frontiers in Psychology, it was shown that listening to Gregorian chanting significantly increased HRV, along with a decrease in cortisol levels, a key marker of stress. HRV represents the variation in time between each heartbeat and is seen as an essential index of vagal tone and the functionality of the parasympathetic nervous system.

Another study by researchers at the University of Pavia in Italy showed that listening to Gregorian chants scored much lower blood pressure, heart rate, and respiratory rate and significantly increased alpha brain wave activity associated with relaxation.

These findings suggest that the soothing, repetitive nature of Gregorian chants is likely to help stimulate the vagus nerve, activate the parasympathetic nervous system, and result in intense relaxation and inner calm.

Chanting Your Way to Inner Peace

So, how do you harness this power of Gregorian chants for Vagus Nerve stimulation and relaxation? Here are a few simple tips to get you started:

1. Find a peaceful and quiet place to sit or lie down.

2. Choose a Gregorian chant that you find attractive. For most people, there are many beautiful options online or on music-streaming services.

3. Just begin to listen to the chants; let the melody flow in your body and mind. Notice how you are feeling or if you perceive anything occurring within your body or mind.

4. As you have began to get comfortable with the frequency chants, then just start to hum or sing along to the frequency chants. You are not meant to know the words or to have a good singing voice—just go for the sound and the vibration.

5. breathe slowly and deeply, letting the belly be full of breath as you inhale and gently soften on the exhale while you are listening or chanting.

6. Practice for 10-20 minutes at a stretch or even longer if you like it.

7. Be patient and consistent. As with any practice, the impact of Gregorian chants on your mind and body may take a while to be noticed. So, try to listen or chant regularly, even for a few minutes each day.

The Gregorian Prescription: Chanting, the Vagus Nerve, and You

As we have learned in this chapter, Gregorian chants provide some of the most potent ancient methods for access to vagal energy and creating deep relaxation and inner calm. Within these hauntingly beautiful melodies, we can rewind the clock of our soul to a timeless place of peace, balance, and resilience in our lives.

Whether you are a lifelong fan of sacred music or new to the world of chant, there has never been a better time to discover the life-transforming power of Gregorian Chants for yourself. Find some quiet time today, put on your favorite recording, and let these ancient melodies do their work on your mind, body, and soul.

So, as you embark on this journey of sonic self-inquiry, keep your approach open, curious, and self-compassionate. Trust that your body and mind know exactly what to do for healing and thriving; through the power of sound and vibration, you are being proactive in your well-being.

And who knows, maybe you would find that missing key to unlock your sense of peace and purpose from the timeless melodies of Gregorian chants.

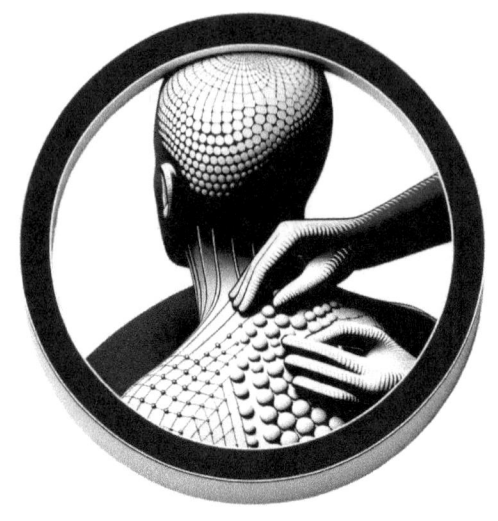

Chapter 8

Acupressure and Massage Techniques for the Vagus Nerve

In this world that seems hurtling along at breakneck speed, it could be easily overlooked how much a simple touch can contribute to our health and well-being. But what if I said you had a powerful tool for balancing your autonomic nervous system, reducing stress, and promoting deep relaxation — all right at your fingertips?

Introduce acupressure and self-massage—two ancient healing arts that work with the time-tested power of touch to stimulate specific points on the body—to release tension and bring back a sense of harmony and flow. These practices tap into the wisdom of traditional Chinese medicine and Ayurveda to form a gentle but powerful way to support our body's healing processes while creating resilience against the stresses of life.

Acupressure, as well as self-massage are both based on the understanding that our human bodies have energy pathways, or meridians, through which the life force moves like rivers from one organ to another. If these pathways are blocked due to overwhelming physical, emotional, and environmental causes or stressors, the consequences would display a variety of symptoms, from pain and tension to anxiety, fatigue, and digestive issues.

The purpose of acupressure and self-massage, then, is based on the assumption that the release of these blockages occurs so that energy is freely flowing and balance is restored within the body. Pressing or massaging key points across these meridians, such as the point of Yin Tang—located between the eyebrows—or the point of Zu San Li, located below the knee, might harness natural healing responses and bring systems back into harmony.

But the benefits of acupressure and self-massage go far beyond mere relaxation. According to research, the practices can go very deep in affecting the autonomic nervous system, which controls functions of heartbeats, digestion, and breathing and is beyond conscious control. Acupressure and self-massage increase relaxation and healing, reduce stress, improve sleep, boost immunity, and promote general well-being by promoting parasympathetic dominance—the "rest and digest" state of the body.

So, what are you waiting for to start using these powerful practices? The beauty of acupressure and self-massage is that both can be done at any time and in any place, with no need for special equipment. All you require are just a few minutes, a quiet place, and the willingness to tune in to your body's subtle cues.

Begin by making yourself comfortably seated or lying, holding a few deep breaths to center yourself. Subsequently, with your fingertips, thumbs, or palms of the hands, rub these regions in your body that usually hold tension, feel sore, or need attention. These could be areas of the feet, hands, neck, or any other part you might need to focus on.

As you work, realize your breath again, allowing your breath to move in and out while your hands are moving. Just surrender to these feelings while trusting that the body is wise and knows exactly what to do to heal and boost the body back up to its optimal level.

Over time, you may also notice a profound change in the physical, mental, and emotional dimensions. You might notice how you become able to sleep more restfully, that your digestion has improved, and that you have a growing sense of profound calm and resilience toward the challenges of life.

So, go ahead and give yourself the gift of touch. Be it a few minutes of self-massage before bed or an entire acupressure session with a practitioner, now that you are tapping into this powerful source of healing and transformation, who knows? You may discover that the key to unlocking your most bottomless vitality and joy has been at your fingertips.

8.1 Craniosacral Therapy and Abhyanga: Soothing the Vagus Nerve through Gentle Touch

Imagine a world in which healing is as simple as lying back, closing your eyes, and letting the power of the gentle touch carry you away. A world in which your most incredible sense of peace and vitality is not out there, in something that is answered, but a wisdom guided from your own body and the skillful hands of a compassionate practitioner.

This is the world of craniosacral therapy and Ayurvedic abhyanga massage—two deep-healing therapies that work with the body's subtle rhythms and energy systems toward creating balance, resilience, and profound relaxation. What lies at the core of this concept is an understanding of the vital role an autonomic nervous system, specifically the vagus nerve, plays in health and well-being.

The vagus nerve, as we've been exploring throughout the book, is like the body's internal compass—a winding path of connection between the brain and gut, heart, lungs, and the rest of the body's most precious organs, and, as such, regulating everything from digestion to heart rate, immune response, and emotional balance. A well-toned and optimally functioning vagus nerve will maintain feelings of calm, connectedness, and resilience in meeting the challenges of living. However when overwhelmed or out of balance as a result of chronic stress, trauma, or other disruptors, it may produce a wide array of bodily and emotional symptoms.

This is where the power of touch comes into play. By working with the subtle rhythms of the body and its energy systems, craniosacral therapy and abhyanga massage provide an extraordinarily gentle and noninvasive way to soothe the vagus nerve, promote parasympathetic dominance, and help a sense of balance and flow be restored to the system.

During a craniosacral therapy session, a therapist would usually apply gentle touch and subtle manipulations while identifying and then releasing the restrictions in the craniosacral system. The practitioner can tap this source by 'listening' to the natural rhythm of the body and guiding this natural process to unlock and facilitate release from any held trauma or tension; hence, it produces a state that is profoundly relaxed and promotes self-healing. This delicate system refers to the network of membranes and fluids that envelop and cushion the brain and spinal cord accessed by touch so gentle in nature. The practitioner, therefore, taps this source by "listening" to the body's natural rhythm and assisting this natural process in unlocking and facilitating release from any held-in trauma or tension, hence creating a profoundly relaxed state promoting self-healing.

Similarly, during the abhyanga massage, beautiful, warm oil is applied to the whole body with long, flowing strokes following the natural energy pathways and nerve endings. According to her, it is a touch full of love, given with aromatic oils, which includes a nourishing touch and rhythmic movement that calms the mind and pleases the senses, creating a deeply felt experience of groundiness and inner peace.

Through either of these practices, the vagus nerve is gently stimulated and soothed, helping to more regulate the autonomic nervous system into a state of poise and ease. Craniosacral therapy and regular abhyanga massage have also been found to improve vagal tone and contribute positively to heart rate variability and other vital markers of autonomic health and resilience.

But maybe even more than the physical benefits are the inroads of profound peace, self-compassion, and integrity that can arise through these practices. Craniosacral therapy and abhyanga massage create a safe, nurturing space for healing and self-discovery. Through these gentle practices, we are spending time without stories and patterns that boundlessly serve us at the deepest level and reconnecting with our inner wisdom and resilience.

They remind us of the power behind the slow, simple, and sacred touch within a world that often feels distracted and pulled apart. They are invitations back home to the self repeatedly and to trust in the profound ability to self-heal and transform.

If you feel called to start exploring the gentle healing arts of craniosacral therapy or abhyanga massage, then know that you are about to begin a journey into profound self-discovery and awakening. Whether you are seeking relief from any physical symptoms, emotional overwhelm, or simply a more profound sense of peace and purpose, these practices offer a portal to the wisdom and completeness that is your birthright.

May you find the courage to step through that doorway in faith for your healing journey, to allow yourself to be held and brought to transformation through the touch of these ancient, sacred practices. May the wafts of the vagus nerve whisk you back home to the most profound truth and beauty of who you are.

8.2 The Ear-Body Connection: Auricular Acupressure and Reflexology for Vagal Tone

Have you ever noticed how massaging or lightly touching the ear makes you feel instantly relaxed, free from tension and stress? This is far from a simple coincidence, as the ear is connected to the entire body through complex nerve lots and important reflex points, including the all-important vagus nerve. By exerting pressure and providing stimulation to particular points on the ears, we can send calming signals to the whole body and thus promote a state of relaxation, balance, and resilience. This is the power of auricular acupressure and ear reflexology.

Auricular acupressure is based on the ancient knowledge of the Chinese medical system – Traditional Chinese Medicine – where the ear is a chart representing the body. Pressing the various points or regions of the ears corresponds to the body's organs and systems, thus causing the body to be treated and balanced easily. For example, the point known as the "Shen Men" or "Spirit Gate" has been said to have a calming effect on the mind and emotions. At the same time, the so-called "Sympathetic" balances the autonomic nervous system and induces relaxation.

Ear reflexology helps to work out the reflex points and zones that interact with various body parts, similar to the more familiar foot reflexology. The softening or pressing of these points allows the energy to travel and brings balance and cure to those parts. For instance, massaging the reflex point for the solar plexus will calm an over-excited sympathetic nervous system, restore a sense of being present, and bring peace.

Possibly the most powerful usage of auricular acupressure and ear reflexology is direct intervention with the vagus nerve, which has one of its branches reaching the ear to connect with the brain and other vital organs. Calming signals may thus be directly sent through this concha or lower cavity of the "vagus point" to the vagus nerve, prompting a state of deep relaxation and recuperation.

So, how do you incorporate auricular acupressure and ear reflexology into your self-care? The easiest way is to apply soft massage or pressure to your vagus point daily for a few minutes, either with fingertips or a small massage tool. Other essential points to consider include Shen Men and the Sympathetic point according to your needs and intentions.

Another effective practice fuses auricular acupressure with deep breathing and mindfulness. So, while massaging or pressing the points, check in with your breath. See if any sensations or emotions come about and allow yourself to be fully present, surrendering to the healing power of your very own touch.

Over time, this kind of practice can lead to profound changes in your nervous system and overall well-being. You will observe that you can step up to stress and increase in challenge with more ease and resilience, and you're feeling more groundedness, centered, and at peace in your daily life.

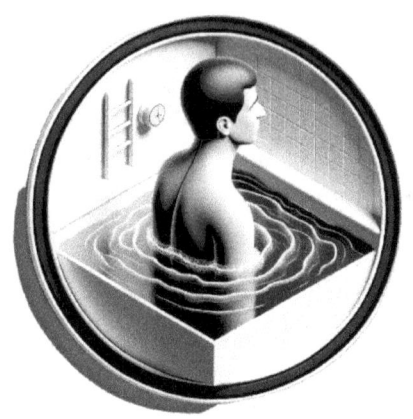

Chapter 9

Cold Exposure and Hydrotherapy for Vagus Nerve Activation

In the realm of health and wellness, a trend is sending chills down our spines – quite literally. Cold exposure, in many forms, has emerged as a key tool for stimulating the vagus nerve, promoting calm, and boosting overall health. From the brisk splash of cold showers to the quiet stillness of ice baths, the power of cold is gaining fame.

But what happens when we face cold? The answer lies in the dance between our autonomic nerves and the vagus nerve. When cold hits the body, it sparks a wave of responses to keep our core warm and aid survival. The first move is a stress response, marked by tight blood vessels, a fast pulse, and stress hormones like norepinephrine.

Yet, as cold exposure goes on, a shift occurs. The "rest and digest" system, led by the vagus nerve, starts to act. This state brings calm, slows the pulse, and eases inflammation. This rebound effect is where the magic of cold exposure lies.

Studies show that cold can boost the vagus nerve, enhancing its tone. This can help balance the nervous system, offering many perks: better heart rate, less inflammation, stronger immunity, improved sleep, and even eased signs of depression and anxiety.

So, how can you harness cold's power? The ways are many, from simple to intense. Cold showers are an easy start, letting you get used to the chill while gaining alertness and better blood flow. For a deeper dive, ice baths or cold plunges give a strong push to the vagus nerve and aid in recovery after hard exercise.

Cryo, with very cold temps (-110°C to -140°C) for short times (2-5 minutes), is now loved by athletes for quick recovery and pain relief. And the old practice of switching between hot and cold, called contrast hydrotherapy, can boost blood flow and cut inflammation.

Even splashing cold water on your face or a cold compress on your neck can trigger the mammalian dive reflex, a response that activates the vagus nerve and brings calm.

As you explore cold exposure, remember to find what fits your body and aims. Start slow, heed your body's cues, and let yourself build tolerance and strength. With patience, you may find that the power of cold unlocks new levels of health, energy, and peace.

9.1 Cold Showers and Ice Baths: Diving into Vagal Tone

Picture this: you stand under a stream of water, ready to start your day. But instead of warm water, you turn the dial to cold. As the icy water hits your skin, you gasp, your heart races, and every nerve in your body comes alive. This is the world of cold showers and ice baths.

While the idea of such cold might seem tough at first, the gains for your health and mood are worth it. Cold showers and ice baths are now popular with health buffs, athletes, and those who want to test their limits. But what happens when you take the plunge?

When you step into a cold shower or ice bath, your body goes through fast changes. The cold triggers a shock: blood vessels shrink, heart rate spikes, and breath quickens. This is driven by the "fight or flight" system.

Yet, as you stay in the cold, a shift happens. Your body starts to adapt, and the "rest and digest" system, led by the vagus nerve, takes over. The vagus nerve helps slow the heart, ease aches, and boost calm.

Cold showers or ice baths can help the vagus nerve and improve health. Studies show cold water boosts heart rate, cuts aches, aids rest, and lifts mood.

How can you start? Go slow and heed your body. For cold showers, start with warm water and slowly lower the temp. Stay in the cold for 30 seconds to 1 minute, focusing on deep breaths. Over time, aim for longer spells.

For ice baths, fill a tub with cold water and add ice until it's 50-59°F (10-15°C). Stay in the water for 10-15 minutes, using deep breaths and calm moves. Always listen to your body and know your limits. If you have health woes, check with a doctor before you dive in.

The benefits of cold showers and ice baths extend far beyond the physical realm. Many people report feeling more energized, focused, and resilient after incorporating these practices into their routines. The mental challenge of facing the cold can help cultivate a sense of inner strength, discipline, and resilience that translates into other areas of life.

So, the next time you're tempted to reach for the warmth of a hot shower, consider embracing the cold instead. By diving into the world of cold showers and ice baths, you're not just giving your vagus nerve a powerful stimulus – you're also tapping into a wellspring of vitality, resilience, and inner peace. Take a deep breath, turn the dial, and let the power of cold transform your body and mind.

9.2 Contrast Therapy and Cold Compresses: Balancing the Autonomic Nervous System

In the broad world of health and care, two strong ways use the chill to balance the body's nerve paths: cold baths and cold packs. These tricks chill parts of the body to wake the vagus nerve, calm the mind, and lift wellness.

Cold baths, known as hydro, use hot and cold water to boost blood flow. The shift in temps helps blood move, cuts swelling, and aids lymph flow. These changes also train the nerve paths, balancing the active and calm sides.

To try a cold bath, soak in hot water (100-105°F) for 3-5 mins to relax muscles and widen blood paths. Then switch to cold water (50-59°F) for 30-60 secs, feeling the paths tighten and the body wake up. Do this 3-5 times, ending with cold for a final boost.

Cold packs, by contrast, target the vagus nerve. A chill pack on the neck or face taps the dive reflex, calming the body. The neck is key, as the vagus runs near the carotid artery. Cooling here can slow the heart, lower blood pressure, and bring calm.

To use a cold pack, soak a cloth in ice water, wring it out, and place it on the neck below the chin. Hold for 2-5 mins, breathing deep. Repeat as needed to calm and relax.

Beyond the vagus, these ways help more. Cold baths aid recovery, ease muscle pain, and boost immunity. Cold packs can ease headaches, cut swelling, and help the gut by sparking the vagus.

Start slow and heed your body. If you have health issues, ask a doctor first. The power lies in the cool feel and the mindful care you bring.

Tune into your body, stay curious and kind to yourself, and embrace the chill. Find a deep well of strength and peace. Fill a bowl with ice, soak a cloth, and give your vagus a cool hug. Your body, mind, and spirit will thank you.

9.2 Embracing the Chill: A Journey of Vagal Nerve Stimulation and Resilience

In this chapter, we've embarked on a journey through the glacial realm of cold exposure, an odyssey that unveils its profound effects on the autonomic nervous system. From cold showers, whose invigorating chill shakes the soul, to ice baths, whose meditative silence freezes time, through the dynamic interplay of contrast therapy and the surgical precision of cold compresses, these practices paint a kaleidoscope of possibilities to awaken the vagus nerve and make well-being blossom.

At the heart of these modalities, pulsating like a heartbeat, thrums a common thread: the deliberate application of cold to unleash a cascade of physiological responses that, like skilled acrobats, balance the nervous system, quell inflammation, and lull the body into relaxation. By challenging our bodies with measured doses of cold stress, we dive into the depths of our innate resilience and adaptability, forging a stronger vagal tone and cultivating a greater sense of equilibrium.

But the benefits of cold exposure extend far beyond the mere physical realm. As we've witnessed, these practices can also cast a profound spell on our mental and emotional well-being, conjuring feelings of vitality, focus, and inner peace. By embracing the discomfort of cold, we learn to face life's challenges with the courage of a warrior and the equanimity of a sage, nurturing a resilience that radiates into every nook and cranny of our existence.

Of course, the path of cold exposure is not always a leisurely stroll. It demands a willingness to step outside our cozy comfort zones, to lean into the discomfort, and to trust in the ancient wisdom of our bodies. It beckons us to cultivate a mindful awareness of our physical sensations and emotional responses, and to approach the practice with the patience of a monk, the compassion of a saint, and the spirit of a curious child.

But for those intrepid souls who dare to brave the chill, the rewards are nothing short of alchemical. By weaving cold exposure into the tapestry of our wellness routines, we not only stimulate our vagus nerves and fortify our physical health – we also tap into a bottomless well of inner strength, resilience, and tranquility.

So, whether you're gingerly dipping your toes into the world of cold showers or plunging headlong into the icy depths of an ice bath, remember that you are embarking on a hero's journey of self-discovery and transformation. Embrace the chill, trust in your body's primal wisdom, and let the power of cold guide you towards a life of exquisite balance, boundless vitality, and unshakable joy.

As you explore the practices outlined in this chapter, approach them with the wide-eyed curiosity of a child, the open-heartedness of a lover, and the self-compassion of a nurturing mother. Start slowly, listen to the whispers of your body's feedback, and celebrate each tiny victory along the way. And remember, the ultimate goal is not merely to endure the cold, but to dance with it – to find within its bracing embrace a wellspring of strength, resilience, and inner peace that will serve as your loyal companion on all the winding paths of your life.

So go ahead, take a deep breath, and plunge into the transformative world of cold exposure. Let the cold be your teacher, your lover, your muse – and watch as your life blossoms into a masterpiece of vibrant health, untamed joy, and limitless possibility.

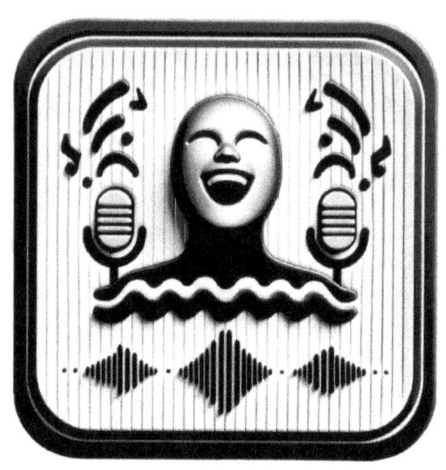

Chapter 10
Laughter, Singing, and Gargling for Vagus Nerve Stimulation

The vagus nerve, the longest nerve in the body, plays a key role in keeping our inner systems in tune, shaping all from heart rate and digestion to how we feel and cope. While there are many ways to wake up the vagus nerve, from deep breathing to cold, some of the most powerful and easy ways use our own voices and mouths.

In this part, we'll look into the amazing world of laughter, singing, humming, chanting, gargling, and even the gag reflex and tongue moves as strong tools for vagus nerve boosts and overall well-being. As we dig into these habits, we'll find out the science behind how they affect the vagus nerve and the inner systems, and give useful tips and ways for adding them into your daily life. Whether you're an old hand at these ways or a curious newbie, this part will give a wealth of ideas and inspiration for using the power of your own voice and mouth to boost health, resilience, and vitality.

So get ready to laugh, sing, hum, chant, gargle, and even stir your gag reflex and do some tongue moves - your vagus nerve (and your entire being) will thank you for it!

10.1 The Healing Power of Laughter and Song

Laughing and singing are two of the most common human acts, going beyond words, ways of life, and age. But more than their power to bring joy and ties, these acts also have a deep impact on our body and mind, mostly due to their effects on the vagus nerve. The Science of Laughing and the Vagus Nerve Laughing is a complex body response that engages many systems in the body, such as the muscles, breathing, and heart. When we laugh, our face muscles move, our breathing changes, and our heart rate and blood flow go up for a bit. But perhaps most key, laughing also wakes up the vagus nerve, turning on the "rest and digest" part of the inner nervous system. This leads to a series of good effects, like:

- Less stress and worry

- More feelings of well-being and social ties

- Better immune work

- Improved heart health

- Better pain control In fact, a study in the Journal of Psychophysiology found that watching a funny film led to more activity in the "rest and digest" part and less activity in the "fight or flight" part of the nervous system in healthy adults, as shown by heart rate changes - a key sign of vagal tone. The Good of Singing for Vagal Tone Like laughing, singing is a strong way to wake up the vagus nerve, thanks to the deep breathing, voice use, and emotions involved. When we sing, several key things happen:

1. Our breath becomes slower and deeper, waking up the vagus nerve through the diaphragm.

2. The shaking made by singing, mostly in the throat and chest, directly wakes up the vagus nerve.

3. The emotions in singing help to control the inner nervous system and boost feelings of well-being.

4. Singing with others helps social bonds and ties, further boosting vagal tone. Research has shown that regular singing can lead to better mood, stress levels, immune work, and even brain skills in older adults. A study in Frontiers in Psychology found that choir singing improved signs of vagal tone, as shown by heart rate changes, and boosted feelings of social ties among those who took

part. Practical Tips for Adding Laughing and Singing So how can you tap into the vagus nerve-boosting power of laughing and singing? Here are some simple tips:

5. Look for humor in your daily life, whether it's watching funny videos, reading jokes, or spending time with people who make you laugh.

6. Try laughing yoga, a way that involves long bouts of on-purpose laughing and deep breathing.

7. Sing in the shower, in the car, or wherever you feel okay letting your voice out.

8. Join a choir or singing group to feel the social benefits of singing with others.

9. Use singing as a way to express emotions, allowing yourself to fully feel and release emotions as you sing. Remember, you don't have to be a pro comic or a trained singer to benefit from these habits. The key is to approach them with a spirit of play, self-kindness, and being open to the experience.

10.2 Humming, Chanting, and Gargling: Simple Yet Powerful Vagus Nerve Hacks

Beyond laughing and singing, there are many other easy ways to wake up the vagus nerve and boost calm, stress resilience, and overall well-being.

These include humming, chanting, and gargling - habits that are easy to learn, need no special gear, and can be done almost anywhere.

The Magic of Humming and Chanting

Humming and chanting are old habits found in many cultures and soul traditions around the world. From Buddhist and Hindu mantras to Native American chants and Gregorian chants, these habits involve saying simple sounds or phrases over and over, often with a certain beat or tone.

The science behind humming and chanting suggests that these habits can have a direct impact on the vagus nerve and the "rest and digest" nervous system. The vibrations made by humming and chanting, mostly in the throat and chest areas, are thought to wake up the vagus nerve, leading to a range of good effects, such as:

- Less stress and worry

- Increased heart rate variability (a sign of vagal tone)

- Better breathing

- Enhanced pain control

- More feelings of calm and well-being

One study in the International Journal of Yoga found that regular "Om" chanting was tied to big drops in stress and worry in healthy people. Another study in Frontiers in Psychology found that humming increased heart rate variability and decreased stress ratings in healthy adults.

Gargling for Vagus Nerve Boosts

Gargling is another simple yet powerful way to wake up the vagus nerve and boost calm and well-being. The act of gargling activates the muscles of the back of the throat, which are connected to the vagus nerve. This boost can lead to a range of good effects, such as:

- Less stress and worry
- Improved heart rate variability
- Better breathing
- More feelings of calm and well-being

In fact, a study in the Journal of Clinical and Diagnostic Research found that daily gargling with warm water was tied to big improvements in vagal tone, as shown by heart rate variability, in healthy adults.

Practical Tips for Humming, Chanting, and Gargling

Ready to try these simple vagus nerve hacks for yourself? Here are some practical tips to get you started:

1. For humming, find a comfy pitch that resonates in your throat and chest. Breathe in deeply, then breathe out while making a long humming sound. Start with a few minutes a day and slowly increase as comfy.

2. For chanting, choose a simple phrase or mantra that feels meaningful to you. Sit comfortably, take a few deep breaths, and begin

saying the phrase over and over, focusing on the feelings of vibration in your throat and chest.

3. For gargling, mix a half teaspoon of salt in a cup of warm water. Take a mouthful, tilt your head back a bit, and gargle for 10-20 seconds. Spit out the water and repeat a few times.

As with any new habit, start slowly and be kind to yourself. Notice any feelings or experiences that come up, without judging. Over time, you may find that these simple ways become valuable tools in your overall wellness toolkit.

Boosting Vagal Tone Through the Gag Reflex and Tongue Moves

Moving deeper into the realm of mouth and face boosts for vagus nerve health, we come to two lesser-known but powerful ways: activating the gag reflex and doing specific tongue moves. While these habits may at first seem odd or even uncomfortable, they are based on a growing understanding of the complex links between the mouth, throat, and inner nervous system.

Waking Up the Gag Reflex for Vagus Nerve Activation

The gag reflex is a protective response that helps prevent choking by triggering the expulsion of objects or substances from the back of the throat. This reflex is controlled by the glossopharyngeal nerve, which is closely tied to the vagus nerve.

Intentionally waking up the gag reflex, such as by using a tongue depressor to gently touch the back of the tongue or throat, has been shown to activate the vagus nerve and promote a range of good effects, such as:

- Increased heart rate variability

- Better digestion and bowel work

- Less inflammation

- Enhanced calm and stress resilience

Of course, it's key to approach gag reflex boosts with care. Always start gently, use a soft, clean tool (like a tongue depressor), and stop if you feel pain or extreme discomfort. It's also key to note that this habit is not recommended for people with a history of eating disorders or severe gag reflex issues.

Tongue Moves for Vagus Nerve Boosts

The tongue is a complex muscle that is connected to many cranial nerves, such as the vagus nerve. Specific tongue moves, sometimes called "orofacial myofunctional therapy," have been shown to wake up the vagus nerve and promote a range of health benefits, such as:

- Better swallowing and speech

- Less snoring and sleep apnea

- Enhanced vagal tone and heart rate variability

- More feelings of calm and well-being

Some simple tongue moves to try include:

1. Tongue Slides: Stick your tongue out and move it slowly from side

to side, holding each position for a few seconds.

2. Tongue Circles: Rotate your tongue around the outside of your lips, first in one direction, then the other.

3. Tongue-to-Nose: Stick your tongue out and try to reach your nose, holding for a few seconds.

4. Tongue-to-Chin: Stick your tongue out and try to reach your chin, holding for a few seconds.

As with gag reflex boosts, start these moves gently and stop if you feel pain. Aim for a few minutes of practice each day, slowly increasing as comfy.

A Note on Safety and Precautions

While the ways described in this section are generally safe for healthy people, it's key to approach them with care and common sense. If you have a history of gagging, choking, or swallowing issues, or if you feel pain or extreme discomfort with any of these habits, stop and check with a healthcare professional before proceeding.

It's also worth noting that while these ways can be powerful tools for vagus nerve boosts and inner balance, they are not a replacement for professional medical care or advice. If you have a serious health condition or concern, please work with a qualified healthcare provider to develop an appropriate treatment plan.

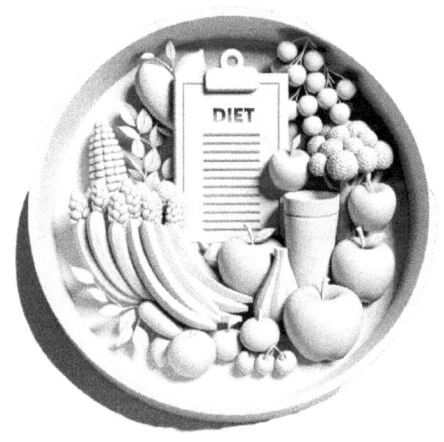

Chapter 11
Nutrition and Diet for Optimal Vagus Nerve Function

Had a "gut feeling" about a thing? Felt "butterflies in your gut" when you were in a bit of stress or joy? These ideas hint at a truth that researchers now grasp: the link between our gut and our mind.

Studies show a strong link between the gut and the mind, known as the gut-brain link. This two-way link includes signals, cells, and nerve paths. One key part of this is the vagus nerve.

The vagus nerve is a long nerve that runs from the brainstem to the gut. It links the brain to many parts of the body, including the gut. This link is not one-way—the vagus nerve serves as a key path for signals between the gut and the mind, with big effects on our health.

In this part, we'll dive into the gut-brain link and see how the vagus nerve acts as a key path in this system. We'll look at new studies on how gut health impacts the vagus nerve and well-being and see some ways to boost this link.

11.1 Nourishing the Gut-Brain Connection

The gut, called our "second brain," has the enteric nerve system (ENS) which works on its own from the main nerve system. But, the gut and brain link via the vagus nerve, letting signals flow both ways, impacting digestion, food take-up, immune action, mood, and acts.

One key role of the vagus nerve in the gut-brain link is to pass sense data from the gut to the brain and modulate gut role and immune action. A fit and mixed gut biome is key for good gut-brain talk and vagus tone. Issues in this fine mix can cause swelling, leaky gut, and even mind and mood woes.

To keep a good gut-brain link, eat a gut-healthy diet rich in fiber, fermented foods, omega-3 fats, and other gut-helpful foods. Manage stress, take aim with added help like probiotics and omega-3s, and use vagus nerve boost ways.

Sarah, age 35, had gut woes and mood dips for months. After she learned about the gut-mind link, she changed her diet, adding more fermented foods, fibers, and omega-3-rich foods. In a few weeks, she saw big gains in her gut health and a more steady, upbeat mood. By feeding her gut-mind link, Sarah boosted her vagus tone and well-being.

11.2 The Power of Fermented Foods and Probiotics

Fermented foods and probiotics are strong tools for a healthy gut biome and good gut-mind link. Probiotics are live bugs that help health when eaten, while prebiotics are foods that help the growth of good gut bugs.

Probiotics help vagus tone by calming the immune system, cutting swelling, and making mood and act signals. Prebiotics give the needed fuel for these good bugs to thrive. Eating both probiotics and prebiotics can help a fit and mixed biome, key for good gut-mind talk and vagus role.

Top foods for probiotics are yogurt, kefir, sauerkraut, kimchi, miso, tempeh, and kombucha. Prebiotic-rich foods are garlic, onions, leeks, asparagus, bananas, oats, and apples. When picking probiotic adds, find a top-notch one with many strains, like Lactobacillus and Bifidobacterium, and third-party checks for purity.

Marcus, age 42, had stress and worry. His guide said to add fermented foods to his diet to help his gut health and vagus tone. Marcus ate kimchi and drank kombucha each day, and took a good probiotic add. After a few months, he felt less worry and more calm. By feeding his gut with fermented foods and probiotics, Marcus helped his vagus nerve and found more calm and strength.

11.3 Maximizing Vagal Tone through the Mediterranean Diet

The Med diet is a way of eating that highlights whole, fresh foods, good fats, and some red wine. The main parts are lots of fruits, greens, whole grains, nuts, and seeds; olive oil; fish, seafood, chicken, eggs, and dairy; and less red meat, junk food, and sugars.

Studies show the Med diet helps heart health, partly by its effects on the vagus nerve and body balance. The good fats and low-swell parts in Med diet foods help heart health, mind work, and well-being by cutting swelling and aiding a fit gut biome.

To use the Med diet, eat plant foods, use good fats like olive oil, eat less meat, enjoy meals with kin and pals, and stay active. This whole way to well-being helps the body, vagus tone, and builds more strength and life.

Elena, age 58, had heart issues in her kin and wanted to care for her heart. She chose the Med diet, eating bright fruits and greens, whole grains, nuts, and good fats like olive oil. Elena also ate with her kin, enjoying the food and bond. After months, her blood tests showed big gains in her heart health. By using the Med way of eating and life, Elena helped her vagus tone, heart health, and felt more well.

11.4 Finding Balance: Caffeine, Alcohol, and Hydration for Optimal Vagal Function

To aim for top health, think about how daily picks impact the body and vagus nerve. Caffeine and alcohol can have mixed effects on vagus health, while water is key to keeping body balance.

Caffeine's effect on the body is tied to dose. Low to mid amounts can boost alertness and mood, but too much can lead to health woes. Some studies say regular, low caffeine use may help vagus tone and heart rate over time. Balance is key—aim for no more than 400 mg a day.

Like caffeine, alcohol's effect is tied to dose and the person. Low to mid amounts can first raise heart rate and cut vagus tone, then lower heart rate and boost vagus tone as alcohol leaves the blood. But, heavy use can lead to health woes. If you drink, aim for low to mid amounts and note your body's signs.

Water is key for body balance and vagus tone. Even slight lack of water can lower heart rate range and raise body stress. To stay well, aim for at least 8 cups of water a day, heed thirst, check urine shade, eat foods with water, limit caffeine and alcohol, and stay cool in heat.

Mike, age 29, liked to stay fit. He wanted to boost his health and performance. He chose to look at his habits with coffee, wine, and water. Mike cut back on his coffee, having just 2-3 cups each day and none late in the day. He also cut down on wine, saving it for big days and staying within safe limits. To stay hydrated, Mike kept a water jug with him, aiming to drink at least 8 cups of water, and checking his urine color to stay well-hydrated.

By balancing his coffee and wine use and making water a priority, Mike helped his vagus tone, boosted his performance, and felt better overall.

As you aim for your best health and well-being, note that what you eat is key for vagus tone and nerve balance. By helping your gut-brain link, using fermented foods and probiotics, eating like in the Med, and balancing coffee, wine, and water habits, you can build more strength, life, and peace. As you start this path, take on each new habit and diet change with care, love, and a goal of listening to your body. With time, effort, and an open heart, you can tap into the full power of your vagus nerve and feel the big gains of a well-fed mind, body, and soul.

Chapter 12
Exercise and Physical Activity or Vagus Nerve Stimulation

The human body is an excellent machine created to move and adapt to the environment's challenges. Nevertheless, many of us remain sedentary in the modern world—being static for long hours behind the desk at work, in the car, or on the sofa at home. This goes a long way in resulting in a lack of physical activity, which has devastating effects on our physical and mental health, contributing to many the chronic diseases and stress-related disorders.

But what if there was one simple, potent way to counteract these effects and promote optimal health and well-being? Enter exercise is the powerful tool to stimulate the vagus nerve and enhance autonomic balance.

As we've been learning throughout this book, the vagus nerve is a critical component of the parasympathetic nervous system, responsible for the body's processes known as "rest and digest." When the vagus nerve is healthy, it supports relaxation, dampens inflammation, and modulates stress responses in the body to support a greater sense of wholeness and resilience.

Research supports that long-term regular exercise favorably affects vagal tone, as reflected by HRV—one of the principal markers of the balance between autonomic components. Routledge et al. (2015) reported that with as little as 12 weeks of moderate intensity, aerobic training marked increases in HRV and general autonomic function could be achieved in previously sedentary adults.

But how does physical exercise affect vagus activity and automatic functioning control? The answer may be found in the complex interplay of physiological and psychological factors.

During exercise, the body undergoes a series of adaptive changes designed to meet the increased demands of oxygen and energy. The "fight or flight" response is activated, and the sympathetic nervous system is excited. This results in increases in heart rate and blood pressure with some increases in respiration. At the same time, the parasympathetic nervous system is momentarily suppressed so that the body can divert its efforts elsewhere.

Regular, moderate physical stress improves autonomic regulation with time. By physically stressing the body using a controlled, progressive overloading approach, exercise could assist in the development of underlying resilience or adaptability—much like a skeletal muscle would be strengthened upon repeated use.

Not only does exercise lead to changes in physiological systems, but the benefits of exercise for vagal tone also cut across powerful effects on mental health and emotional well-being, all closely connected to autonomic function.

It has been shown to alleviate the symptoms of anxiety and depression, improve cognitive functioning and memory, and enhance self-efficacy concerning stress resilience. Some, but not all, of these gains in psychological well-being are assumed to be mediated by the release of neurotransmitters such as serotonin, dopamine, and endorphins, which help in mood stabilization and the development of well-being.

Furthermore, exercise may provide mindfulness and body awareness in individuals, where one can listen to his body's signals and develop a higher level of presence and self-regulation. Learning to listen to the body's signals and responding to them with care and compassion will anesthetize a higher degree of mind-body integration and autonomic balance.

So how can you start using more movement throughout your day to help vagal tone and overall health? The good news is that there are countless ways to get active. From walking and jogging to dancing and martial arts, the list goes on. You just need to find what you enjoy, which provides a challenge yet feels doable and sustainable over the long run.

Here are some pointers to consider:

1. Start small and build gradually: If you are a novice to exercising, start with short, manageable bouts of activity that gradually increase in intensity and duration.

2. Consistent Routine: The benefits of exercise on vagal tone are cumulative; therefore, it is essential to include physical activity as part of one's routine and not as a one-off activity.

3. Mix it up. Combine the best of aerobic, strength, and mind-body types of exercise, like yoga and Tai Chi, so there is some cross-sectional workout that stimulates both mind and body.

4. Listen to your body: It's also important to push yourself, but at the same time, treat your body right and don't overtrain or push through pain or injury.

5. Socialize: One can be able to involve friends, family, or any other group that is affiliated with you in the practice of exercises since it will provide motivation, sharing accountability, and a sense of connection among them for support.

Remember, it's not about the perfect movement; it's the progressive realization of adding more movements into your daily life. So, with every move you make, you walk a little closer to health, resilience, and vibrancy.

Lace-up your shoes, find a buddy, head out, and keep moving. Your vagus nerve (and your whole body) will thank you.

12.1 Aerobic and Resistance Training: A Powerful Combination for Vagal Health

Whereas any physical activity appears to bless the vagal tone and autonomic balance, two peculiar ways emerge more consistently in the literature as having potent effects on vagal function: aerobic exercise and resistance exercise.

Cardio exercise, more commonly known as "aerobic exercise," is any rhythmic sustained activity that increases both heart and breathing rate. An example includes such exercises as walking, jogging, cycling, or swimming, which put the cardiovascular and respiratory systems under a particular strain and make them get used to supplying the body's tissues with more oxygen and nutrients. Over time, a plethora of health benefits can be expected.

Studies have consistently shown that regular aerobic exercise leads to improvements in heart rate variability (HRV) and vagal tone, particularly in previously sedentary individuals. For example, a meta-analysis by Sandercock et al. (2005) found that aerobic exercise increased the HRV with an effect that was more pronounced in older adults and those with lower baseline levels of fitness.

Besides physical fitness, the benefits of aerobic exercise are derived from a better vagal tone. There are potent influences of regular cardio exercise on mental health and emotional well-being; it lowers depression and anxiety and creates a more resilient and self-effective individual toward stress (Sharma et al., 2006).

Some of the psychological benefits of aerobic exercise could be suggested to be mediated via the effects of the latter on the brain's neurotransmitter systems, specifically serotonin, and norepinephrine, both of which play essential roles in the regulation of mood and stress responses.

Resistance training, on the other hand, involves the manipulation of weights, machines, or body weight as a form of challenge to make muscles more robust and more resilient. It has often been equated to muscular mass and strength building; however, resistance training has also been shown to impact autonomic function and vagal tone significantly.

A 12-week resistance training program in postmenopausal women with hypertension found significant improvements in HRV and baroreflex sensitivity. The authors suggested that the increased muscle strength and endurance produced by resistance training may improve vagal tone through a reduction in sympathetic activity and promotion of parasympathetic dominance.

Other evidence supports that resistance training can have positive effects on bone density, insulin sensitivity, and cognitive function, important for overall health and well-being of an aging population (Westcott, 2012).

So, how should you combine both cardiovascular and resistance training in a session to maximize the benefits to vagal tone and autonomic balance?

Here's some advice:

1.Use complementary exercise: Both aerobic and resistance training exercises are helpful, so it is better to make a mixture of both in the routine instead of having a focus on only one type.

Start with the basics: If you are a newcomer to exercise, start with simple, foundational movements like body squats with your weight, pushups, and rowing exercises.

3. Proper Form: Proper technique is essential to gain the best benefit from resistance training and injury reduction. Working with a qualified trainer or coach on form and progression would be appropriate.

4. Push yourself: To keep making progress in not only strength but also vagal tone, the intensity and complexity of your workouts have to go up slowly over time—but always listen to your body and be careful of overtraining.

5.Recover and rest: Sufficient rest and recovery between workouts are critical to providing time for the body to adapt and, hence grow stronger. You should be looking to get at least one day of complete rest per week. Pour sweat, not too much, and ensure ample sleep and stress management as part of your general training strategy.

Just as you learn to work with both aerobic and resistance exercises, remember that the journey toward increased strength, resiliency, and balance of the autonomic nervous system is a process; it's not a goal that you have to reach with all speed. Be patient with yourself. Celebrate your progress and trust that each step you take toward further physical activity is a step toward a more vibrant, challenging, and rewarding life.

12.2 Mind-Body Practices: Cultivating Vagal Tone through Yoga, Tai Chi, and Nature Walks

These two exercises are great, no doubt, in enhancing vagal tone and autonomic balance. Still, there are many other ways toward more excellent health and resilience that are more complementary than alternative, supporting vagal function in sub-serving this relationship among the physical, mental, and emotional aspects of our being: other meditative, mind-body practices such as yoga or Tai Chi, or even nature walks.

Yoga is an ancient Indian philosophical and spiritual practice representing a natural system of physical postures, techniques of breathing, and training of reflection to provide harmony, flexibility, and inner peace. Over time, many researchers have ascertained that the systematic practice of yoga brings significant changes in autonomic function, resulting in the reduction of sympathetic activity and an increase in parasympathetic tone (Tyagi & Cohen, 2016).

It is believed that one of the primary mechanisms by which yoga can help to support vagal function is through the focus on deep, diaphragmatic breathing. Most yogic activities are associated with slow, controlled breathing, such as in pranayama, and some asanas that make an individual breathe to their diaphragm, hence stimulating the vagus nerve in a manner that brings about relaxation and emotional control (Brown & Gerbarg, 2005).

This can be heightened to include mindfulness and body awareness through yoga and, thus, may help people develop greater self-regulation and resilience concerning stress and challenge. He can learn how to carefully observe and accept the thoughts and feelings that arise, together with the physical sensations and reactions, in a compassionate and non-judgmental way toward himself to develop that sense of inner peace and emotional balance (Khattab et al., 2007).

An ancient Chinese practice, Tai Chi combines gentle, flowing, slow-motion movement with breath awareness and meditation. The ancillary benefits of these practices are significant effects on autonomic function and vagal tone, much like yoga does. They emphasize the mind-body integrative cultivation of inner balance through slow, graceful movements combined with focused attention; in other words, relaxing and reducing stress.

Studies have shown that regular practice of Tai Chi and Qigong can change heart rate variability, baroreflex sensitivity, and other markers of autonomic function in particular among older practitioners and those with chronic conditions, chronic diseases, or postoperative conditions including injury to the autonomic nervous system. These practices have also been found to be effective about mental health and emotional well-being, reducing the symptoms of anxiety and depression and promoting a greater sense of vitality and self-efficacy (Wang et al., 2010).

For my part, walking in nature is perhaps one of the easiest and most potent ways of nurturing vagal tone and, in turn, inner harmony. We, as humans, have walked on this Earth for a million years near nature. Our minds and bodies are attuned to the patterned rhythmic cycles of the Earth.

A burgeoning body of research over the past decade has provided consistent evidence that exposure to nature, or more precisely when involved in modest, rhythmic activities like walking, influences autonomic function and emotional state. For example, Park et al. (2010) showed that a 15-minute walk in a forest environment had a significantly greater heart rate variability and parasympathetic activity than an urban walk.

Additionally, feeling nature sensually—for example, the sounds of the birds and the trees, the sun on the skin, and the earth beneath one's feet—can also place someone in the present moment, leading to mindfulness and inner peace. This lets people plug off the surroundings that might stress and distract them and get down to the beauty and simplicity of nature in a way that fosters greater connection, gratitude, and awe.

How to start using these mind-body practices to get your vagal tone and inner balance supporting your life:

1. Begin with curiosity: Do not practice these practices as if it is another rule-based perfectionism, instead have a spirit of being curious with them. Let yourself be interested, and feel free to play with the styles and techniques until you find the ones that sound good to you.

2. Make it a practice: Like any skill, developing vagal tone through mind-body practices takes time and effort. Work toward a commitment to doing these in some organized way each day or week—even for a few minutes at a time.

3. Find a community: Take your yoga or Tai Chi or walk into the community when you can. This should encircle you with a sense of connection, support, and accountability that, then, you can mirror with local classes or

groups or by inviting friends and family to join in with you on what you do.

4. Incorporate into daily routine: Find ways to weave these practices into your daily routine. A few deep breaths before a stressful meeting, a quick round of Tai Chi while waiting in line, or a short nature walk during lunch.

5. Stay patient and compassionate: Remember that the journey toward greater tone and inner balance is lifelong, not a destination. Be patient with yourself and celebrate your progress along the way; extend compassion and kindness to yourself when you stumble or fall short.

Once you finally start to implement them in your life, remember that, in essence, you are building one of the most valuable internal resources for these life challenges and insecurities. With each deep breath, each mindful movement, and each step taken in nature, you strengthen your vagal tone, resilience, and capacity for joy, connection, and inner peace.

Therefore, pause for a while and tune in to your breathing; feel your chest rise and fall, air moving in and out of your lungs. And with every passing moment, learn that you're gaining an even more profound sense of presence, balance, and wholeness, which will serve you well on the journey ahead.

Near the end of this chapter, as we roll toward exercise and physical activity relative to vagus nerve stimulation, it seems only fitting that for a moment, we stand back and wonder at the beautiful power movement possesses to keep us healthy, strong, and well.

From the physiological adaptations of aerobic and resistance training to the mind-body integration of yoga, Tai Chi, and nature walks, the practices and principles we have been considering in this chapter offer a multifaceted approach to supporting vagal tone and autonomic balance. Regular physical and mind-body activities develop the inner resources of resilience and invite one to develop a more profound sense of connectedness to one's physical, mental, and emotional self—thus learning to thrive amidst life's challenges.

But perhaps the most essential message that underlies the practices and principles of the chapter we have just explored is that they call us back to a sense of joy, playfulness, and curiosity in relationship with our movement and bodies. Too often, exercise has come to be viewed as a necessity, or worse, a punishment, something we "should" do to compensate for our perceived failings or limitations. But what if we moved in wonder, with gratitude toward the body and with compassion toward ourselves? What if we found things from that place that nourished and enlivened us, that made us feel more alive, connected, and whole?

As you go along to better vagal tone and autonomic balance, exercise and physical activity the same spirit of curiosity, play, and self-discovery. Try a new way of moving the body: dance, hike, martial arts, team sport—or whatever way. Note your body and mind's reactions to different activities and be naturally attracted to those that bring exhilaration, energy, and peace.

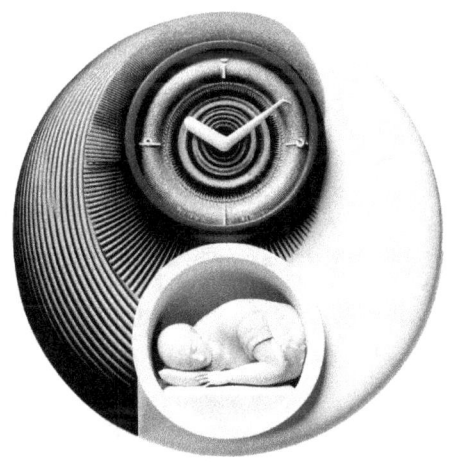

Chapter 13
Sleep and Circadian Rhythm or Vagus Nerve Health

In the jigsaw of our health and well-being, sleep is the critical piece that knits the physical, mental, and emotional realms of our lives together. Not only is it an essential period of rest and rejuvenation, but it is also equally a multifaceted, dynamic process key to the full optimal functioning of the body and the brain.

At the core of the process lies the autonomic nervous system, and at the center of the autonomic nervous system regulating our sleep-wake cycles and maintaining balance and the state of resilience is the vagus nerve. The vagus nerve is part of the parasympathetic nervous system. It reshapes the "rest and digest" functions of the body, telling it to relax, lower inflammation, and favor the other natural sleep-and-heal processes.

It has been established that sleep deprivation significantly influences the reduction in vagal tone, an index of autonomic balance and resilience, as measured by heart rate variability (HRV). Chronic sleep deprivation has been related to a gamut of adverse health consequences like impaired immunity, increased inflammation, hormonal imbalances, reduced pain tolerance, and impaired cardiovascular function.

Alternately, optimal quality sleep and maintaining a consistent sleep pattern positively impact vagal tone and overall health and well-being. Plenty of sleep allows one to enter a state of profound parasympathetic dominance, in which the vagus nerve can work its restorative magic to trigger both physical and emotional healing.

Good sleep hygiene and sleep-friendly preparations are designed to support healthy sleep and vagal function. This can be helped by regular waking and sleeping time, having a soothing pre-sleep routine, ensuring the sleeping environment is comfortable, and keeping stress under control.

As a hard-working marketing executive, Julia had always considered sleep deprivation a badge of honor; she could burn the midnight oil with the best of them. Over time, though, she started to realize the impact that chronic sleep deprivation was having on her health and well-being. She was plagued by a constant string of colds, mood swings, and a generalized sense of fatigue that no amount of caffeine could remedy.

She didn't even try to get to bed in the same timely way until she learned that it's part of great vagal tone. She first started by creating a consistent bedtime and wake time, established a calming bedtime routine with such activities as brushing her teeth, putting on her pajamas, taking a warm bath, and drinking calming chamomile tea, and then optimized her sleep environment for great slumber.

As Julia started placing more importance on her sleep, she began to experience fundamental changes in her physical and emotional balance: she noticed her immune system picking up again, her mood beginning to even out, and, most importantly, she now had so much more energy and focus during the day. I also found that the grip of stress and challenges was better managed at work and in my personal life.

Julia's is a true story, pointing to how transformational sleep can be for our health and well-being. By honoring this most central tenet of self-care, we tap into the healing power of the vagus nerve, cultivating balance, resilience, and vitality through the rest of our lives.

As we navigate our ways through modern living, it is high time that we highly value and give as a gift to ourselves sleep and set time sacredly for reconnection in our daily schedules. Utilizing the natural rest our body solicits, paired with the power of the vagus nerve, we can lay the groundwork for a life of greater vitality, resilience, and joy.

13.1 Circadian Rhythms, Vagal Function, and Holistic Health

In the large-scale orchestra of our bodily systems, the circadian rhythm emerges as a master conductor guiding the goings on and off of innumerable physiological processes. This 24-hour internal clock, fine-tuned over millions of years of evolution, coordinates such things as sleep-wake cycles, the release of hormones, and the regulation of body temperature and metabolism to ensure our body functions well, in the best possible way, in synchrony with the natural rhythms of day and night.

Interestingly, the circadian rhythm is very intricately associated with the function of the vagus nerve, which happens to be the most prolonged and most complex of the cranial nerves. Serving as an interface of communication between the central circadian pacemaker in the brain and peripheral organs, it is a significant mediator of synchronization and regulation of biological rhythms.

Research has also found that disturbances of circadian rhythmicity—be they provoked by shift work, jet lag, or irregular sleep—have severe impacts on vagal function and, consequently, health. Chronic circadian misalignment has been associated with reduced heart rate variability as a marker of decreased vagal tone and autonomic imbalance. The latter has been linked to various metabolic dysfunctions, cardiovascular disease, and mood disorders.

Additionally, circadian rhythm disruptions may affect the production and secretion of melatonin, a hormone closely associated with vagal function and sleep regulation. Its reduction has been linked to disturbed sleep, metabolic disturbances, and low immune response.

Aligning our internal clocks with the natural light-dark cycle and decreasing our exposure to predictors of the day-night cycle disruptors would ensure our rhythms and vagal tone remain pretty intact. These would presumably include keeping a regular sleep-wake schedule, maximizing light exposure to natural outdoor light during the day, and minimizing light exposure, particularly that of artificial lighting, at night.

Marcus was a long-haul truck driver who had accustomed himself to the erratic sleep patterns and long stretches of night driving that came with his job. He had just started suffering from a slow decline in health and well-being, experiencing constant fatigue, digestive disturbances, and a chronic feeling of being out of sync.

Marcus was able to understand this fact only after he had learned that the vagal function is related to the functioning of circadian rhythms. He started making small but consistent changes to his routine, including trying to sleep regularly whenever possible, getting as much natural light as possible during the day, and winding down his bedtime routine with meditation and deep breathing exercises.

Though sometimes hard to keep up in the field, Marcus learned that orienting his energy around circadian health made a monumental difference in how he felt. He noticed more energy, his digestion, and mood improved; he felt more robust under pressure and the vagaries of his boss's job.

Marcus's experience, by contrast, points heavily to the significant importance of developing an awareness of and respect for our internal rhythms in light of the demands and distractions of contemporary life. In aligning our life with these natural cycles of lightness and darkness, we tap into a deep resource of balance, resilience, and vitality—key ingredients vitally crucial for the optimal functioning of our Vagus Nerve and, really, of our general health.

It is the ultimate self-care and self-empowerment act of becoming conversant with the intelligence of our circadian rhythms and endorsing vagal tone using simple yet powerful lifestyle changes in this disconnected world from the natural world. By attuning ourselves to the subtleties of the body and the world, we awaken into this more profound sense of connection, harmony, and flow, which can guide us to more fantastic realms of health, happiness, and purpose.

13.2 Vagal Tone and the Art of Napping

When it comes to sleep and restoration, The power of a nap is underestimated and a kind of luxury reserved for the very young or very old. Nevertheless, strategic napping can help contribute to vagal tone, cognitive function, and even well-being in conditions of sleep deprivation and the challenge of circadian rhythm.

Power napping, taking a short sleep in the daytime, has been proven to accrue vaunted benefits to autonomic function and vagal tone. Studies show that napping for 20–30 min leads to increased heart rate variability, a quantitative measure of vagal tone, and an indirect measure of autonomic balance. While the short time frame for a nap will likely lead to changes toward a more relaxed and restorative state, parasympathetic dominance may be more supportive of health and well-being.

However, naps can be vastly enhanced or detrimental by when, how long, and how frequently they are taken. For example, napping too late in the day has the potential to eat into nighttime sleep and, as such, interferes with the sleep-wake schedules, resulting in a feeling of confusion and highly groggy. Taking too much time napping can also lead to sleep inertia, a depressive state of waking with a reduction in cognitive function and a state of low alertness, usually for some minutes to hours.

Optimize the benefit of napping for vagal tone and overall well-being by scheduling naps of short duration (20-30 minutes) in the early afternoon when circadian rhythms dip and sleepiness visits.

Furthermore, the environment in which the napping should be done is accommodative and comfortable, such as being quiet and dark, with limited interference, to assist the napper in deriving the best restorative ability from the practice. Some people may do well with relaxation techniques, like deep breathing and progressive muscle relaxation exercises, to be helped into a restful state.

Sarah, an undergraduate student with an overwhelming course load combined with part-time employment, for long, has been a setting sun to napping at any time, considering it a weakness or laziness. But with increasing demands from the schedule slowly cannibalizing her sleep and quality regularly, she decided to give strategic napping a try.

From that point, she began borrowing 20-30 minutes of the early afternoon to slip a brief nap into a quiet, darkened room. She would set the alarm so as not to oversleep and to keep naps on a regular schedule, even when she thought she might power through an afternoon.

Surprisingly, such brief strategic interludes in the day indeed seemed to make a difference for her in having higher supplies of energy, a better mood, and her brain functioning. She had much more alertness and focus during her afternoon classes and work shifts, was much better at handling stress with balance, and had a perspective that allowed her to navigate her busy schedule.

Sarah's experience hints at the potential power that napping could prove to be in supporting vagal tone and general well-being, particularly under conditions of sleep deprivation or circadian disruption. Intention, strategy, and greater awareness allow us access to this significant source of rest and restoration, which will vary between people and help us stay resilient and graceful in the face of challenges and requirements in life.

Of course, sleep is not one-size-fits-all, and what works for one person may not work for another. Some people may feel groggy and disoriented for a while after the nap, while others can face disadvantages in falling asleep at night.

The key is to look at napping with a sense of curiosity and an awareness of your self by paying attention to how such a practice impacts your energy levels, mood, and overall well-being. Proceeding with a spirit of flexibility and experimentation as to when and where your nap is open, so you can change and adapt as you learn what works well for your needs.

It has much to do with napping rather than just snatching a few minutes more of sleep. In other words, it is about developing this more profound sense of attunement and responsiveness to the natural rhythms and needs of your own body and affording those moments of rest and respite in a world that finds most of its activities and demands for productivity almost incessant.

As we all navigate our way through the twisted challenges of modern life, napping may just be a game-changer in self-care and self-compassion for all of us, putting us in remembrance of the wisdom behind the body's innate need for rest and recovery. The more we gain access to this strategic restorative power by using napping, the more we support better vagal tone, health, and well-being in general, and the more we can show up fully in our lives rather than partially.

13.3 Supporting Vagal Tone through Natural Sleep Aids and Lifestyle Practices

An attempt to secure sleep restoration and optimize vagal tone will inexorably involve natural sleep remedies and lifestyle practices that enable the body's healing drive and support general health and well-being. From nature-derived medications such as herbal extracts and supplements to mindfulness methods and environmental changes, there are many ways available to elicit the shift into a quiet, safe state and trigger the activity of the vagus nerve.

Among natural sleep aids, one of the most studied is melatonin. It is an endogenous hormone that regulates sleep-wake cycles. Many studies have shown that supplementary melatonin improves the quality and quantity of sleep, particularly in persons with jet lag, shift work disorder, and other circadian rhythm sleep disorders. Melatonin potentially possesses anti-inflammatory and antioxidant activity, supporting increased vagal tone.

Other natural sleep aids are considered in terms of their ability to soothe, relieve stress and anxiety, and contribute to better sleep. Compounds like valerian root, magnesium, L-theanine, and lavender act at multiple biological mechanisms: modulating the activity of brain neurotransmitters, relaxing muscles, and inducing calmness or tranquility.

Although they may be effective in supporting sleep and vagal tone, natural sleep aids must be used with a great deal of caution, guided by the healthcare provider, since some of them test negatively in interaction with other medications or may have unwanted side effects, especially when taken in large quantities and for a more extended period.

Besides natural sleep aids, lifestyle practices and environmental modifications can go a long way in the restoration of proper healthy sleep and support of vagal function in the body. These include: setting a regular sleep schedule, establishing pre-sleep rituals, designing the sleep environment, using active muscle relaxation, avoiding intake of caffeine and alcohol, engaging in exercise, and managing stress and anxiety.

Ethan was a thirty-five-year-old software engineer who stayed awake all night. He liked to work at night, and because of this, he kept on waking up very groggy and unrefreshed. He would try to counteract this with all kinds of creative ideas and caffeine and sugary snacks throughout the day.

Then, when Ethan started feeling much more anxious and, over time developed excessive digestive disorders, he realized it was high time to work on his sleep habits and to study natural support for health and well-being. He set a consistent bedtime and wake time and established a relaxing bedtime routine with stretching, reading books, journaling, and following an optimized bedroom environment with comfortable bedding, blackout curtains, and a white noise machine.

Ethan also tried natural sleep-inducing agents, such as melatonin and valerian root, and stress-alleviating practices, like deep breathing and mindfulness meditation, in his daily routine. He found that the combination of lifestyle changes and targeted supplementation had a noticeable impact on his relaxation, sleep, stress relief, energy levels, and overall well-being.

Ethan, the holistic psychologist, mentioned that after he had begun to prioritize his sleep and well-being, he found that many things in his physical and mental health changed. The symptoms of anxiety became less and less frequent and less painful; digestion improved; resilience and adaptability to the challenges at work and in life were felt. Also, he could observe that he was capable of thinking much more straightforward and communicating much better, which brought more presence and engagement in his personal and professional relationships.

What emerges from Ethan's story is illustrative of the highly transformative potential of natural systems involved in sleep and lifestyle practices that support vagal tone and overall health. In this way, a holistic, multi-faceted approach to sleep and self-care nurtures the body's ability to heal itself and build more balance, resilience, and vitality back into our lives.

Of course, what works for one person doesn't work for the next, so natural sleep aids and changes in lifestyle should be approached with lots of curiosity, patience, and self-compassion. This can require time and some experimentation to get the combinations of strategies that work best for your unique needs and circumstances. There can be hitches and bumps along the way to your goal; after all, everything in life doesn't just go smoothly.

The point is to remain open, flexible, and committed to self-discovery and self-care, believing in small, consistent changes that will accumulate over time for significant changes in sleep, health, and overall well-being.

Supporting vagal tone with these nature-based sleep aids and lifestyle practices is about something much more foundational than good sleep. It's about cultivating deeper attunement and alignment with the profound wisdom and healing capacities of your body and creating the conditions for excellent health, happiness, and flourishing in all areas of life.

At a time when we press forward with more and more ways to overcome the challenges and complexities of the modern world, getting back to the basics of natural empowerment through healing and self-care could be the most radical act of resilience: a continuing reminder to respect the needs of our bodies, minds, and spirits as we tend to the delicate autonomic nervous system underpinnings that provide the foundation for our overall health and well-being.

It is this kind of sleep that prioritizes nourishing our vagal tone, in which calm, ease, and flow are cultivated during the daily process, opening the portal to a life rich in more vitality, creativity, and connection, and to the unlimited potential to live in a way that is congruent with our deepest values and aspirations.

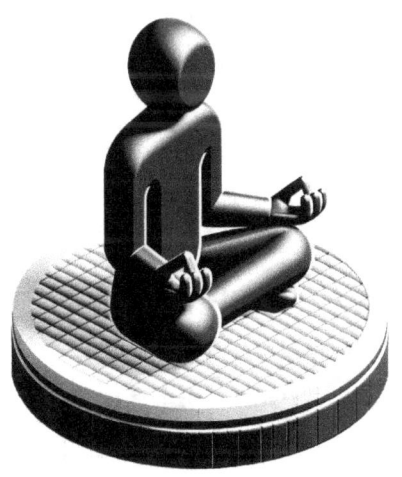

Chapter 14
Stress Management and Relaxation Techniques for Vagal Tone

Stress becomes a familiar companion in the crazed, fast, dynamic globalization of our existence. Is it little, inconsequential rigmaroles of everyday living or great adversity that strikes like the hammer of Thor during significant life events; stress has its snowy effect on physical, mental, and emotional well-being.

The vagus nerve is part of the autonomic nervous system but becomes very important when we discuss the management of stress by the body. The vagus nerve is critical in promoting relaxation—by decreasing inflammation and increasing overall health—in a healthy functional state. Chronic stress may bring a dysregulation in the function of the autonomic nervous system, with a host of adverse health consequences resulting.

Research indicates that chronic stress tends to reduce vagal tone, as picked up by heart rate variability. Reduced HRV has been associated with cardiovascular disease, depression, and many, many other diseases. Other effects include chronic stress that leads to gastrointestinal complaints, immunosuppression, dysregulation of the hormonal system, accelerated senescence, undermined capacities for cognition, and impaired social engagement.

Chronic stress also affects the psyche, increasing the likelihood of anxiety, depression, and burnout. Dysregulating the vagus nerve as a consequence of chronic stress might lead it into a vicious cycle, making it, with time, progressively harder for the organism to relax and come back to a balanced state.

Effectively managing stress promotes optimal vagal tone and overall well-being. The use of relaxation and healthy lifestyle habits allows us to support vagus tone in naturally regulating stress so that we can be resilient.

Here are some effective strategies for managing stress:

1. Deep breathing practice tends to stimulate the vagus nerve and produce a relaxation response.

2. Exercise regularly to reduce stress and maintain good autonomic system function.

3. Add some mindfulness and meditation to quiet the mind and soothe anxiety.

4. The main concern here is good quality sleep, which allows the body to heal and restore body functions naturally.

5. Nurturing supportive social connections to foster a sense of belonging and emotional well-being.

It used to be that Emily, with her fast-rising corporate lawyer career, would get her adrenaline fix in the fast world of law. With each passing year, however, she realized how the chronic stress was increasingly taking a toll on her health. She would have splitting headaches, digestive problems, and an utter feeling of fatigue constantly.

It was only after she learned that vagal tone was linked to stress that Emily worked on the critical area of stress management in her life. Much of it was focused on daily deep breathing exercises and mindfulness practices, exercise, and time for social engagements.

As Emily started to take care of herself, she realized the massive difference she was experiencing in her physical and mental health. The headaches and indigestion she had been battling were starting to fade away. Emily was beginning to feel better in her general energy, leading to a new level of resilience during stress. She even found out that her relationships and her work performance were significantly improved by maintaining an increased balance and presence.

These are just a few examples of how Emily's story is a compelling reminder of how excellent change stress management makes to one's health and well-being. We are therefore supporting the vagus nerve's overall most excellent capacity in regulating stress for the attainment of excellent health by providing ourselves with the best support possible in relaxation and self-care.

14.1 Mastering the Art of Relaxation: Diaphragmatic Breathing and Progressive Muscle Relaxation

There have been proven relaxation techniques powerful and well proven in stress management for the support of vagal tone—diaphragmatic breathing and progressive muscle relaxation, or PMR. It is a simple yet powerful technique that is able to elicit relaxation within the body, reducing tension and activating the vagus nerve.

It involves using the diaphragm, the large muscle at the base of the lungs, to take slow and deep breaths. This mode of breathing allows for a better exchange of oxygen and carbon dioxide, which subsequently leads to deep relaxation and a reduction in stress.

For practicing diaphragmatic breathing, sit comfortably and place one hand on your chest and the other on your belly. Inhale slowly and deeply through your nose, directing your breath into your stomach so you feel it push your hand out. Exhale slowly through puckered lips, feeling your belly retreat towards your spine. Do this for a few minutes, paying attention to the sensation of your breath leaving and entering your body.

It is stated that the regular practice of diaphragmatic breathing increases heart rate variability—a marker of healthy vagal tone—and reduces symptoms of stress, anxiety, and depression. Diaphragmatic breathing helps promote relaxation that ultimately helps stimulate the parasympathetic nervous system, which is an excellent tool in stress management and well-being.

Research has shown that progressive muscle relaxation systematically involves tensing and relaxing various muscle groups of the body, thus giving a deep sense of relaxation and releasing physical tension. If you guide someone through the process of tension and release in each muscle group, PMR will typically help to simply calm their mind, and it will help induce a feeling of inner peace.

To practice PMR, find a comfortable position and take a few deep breaths. The toes and the undersides of your feet are tensed very slightly, gently. Hold for 5-10 seconds and release, letting the muscles go completely. A little later, bring your attention gradually through the muscles of your body, first focusing on the calves, then thighs, then on through the neck and face, tensing progressively a little more and then releasing each muscle group, one by one.

As does diaphragmatic breathing, PMR offers manifold advantages to the mind and body: a decrease of muscle tension, a decrease of stress and anxiety, improved HRV, enhanced immune system function, and better quality of sleep. Inducing a deep state of relaxation and releasing physical tension, PMR can be a great addition to other techniques used for stress management.

Sophie, a mother of three grown children, has always been busy. With three kids and running her small business, Sophie was, as expected, overwhelmed and exhausted all the time. It wasn't until she discovered the power of diaphragmatic breathing and PMR that she began to find a sense of inner calm and balance.

Sophie started her day by focusing on her belly, riding the swell as it filled with air, and then allowing her diaphragm to relax for three minutes of diaphragmatic breathing. She used PMR in bed at night in much the same way to become drowsy.

With daily practice of these skills, Sophie came to experience a massive change in well-being and stress management. She felt balanced, strong, and clear so that she could go forward in her life, her work, and her relationships.

Sophie's story illustrates how diaphragmatic breathing and PMR dynamically change the tools available for stress management and influence the support of vagal tone. Doing it regularly feels peaceful but rugged and healthy when times are hard.

14.2 Using the Power of Your Mind: Guided Imagery, Visualizations, and Relaxation Exercises

Beyond bringing about physical relaxation methods for relieving or decreasing stress, the mind can also be asked to help promote the vagal tone. Guided imagery, visualization, and personalized relaxation routines enable the creation of inner quietness and a lessening of stress for general well-being.

Guided imagery and visualization can tap into the power of the mind in constructing full-sensory experiences toward relaxation and positive emotions. Activate the senses to an experience in which everything seems as though it is happening for the process of helping activate the body's relaxation response and stimulating the vagal nerve.

Guided imagery and visualization have also been shown to be effective in improving a variety of other physical and mental health-related symptoms, such as decreased stress and anxiety, strengthened immunity, enhancement of pain management skills, and improvement in sleep and emotional regulation. These skills can further deepen relaxation and positive imagery proving to be significant stress management skills that enhance vagal tone.

For guided imagery or visualization, locate yourself in a quiet and comfortable place and take a few deep breaths. Begin by focusing on your goal for this relaxation, such as calming or releasing tension. Then, let your imagination construct a very detailed experience of being there, perhaps actually walking along a beautiful beach or hiking through a peaceful forest. Engage all your senses and be there: see, hear, smell, and feel your imagined world. Just let yourself fully enter the experience and let go of all those bothersome thoughts and worries.

Here is where the development of a personalized relaxation regimen can also be a powerful way of showing that stress management is a high priority and of supporting vagal tone, besides guided imagery and visualization. A few minutes daily for the practice of relaxation will counterbalance the toll that stress levies on the body, thereby developing a more excellent balance and resiliency.

Feel free to add it any techniques that you find especially compelling or that are comfortable for you, whether it be deep breathing, progressive muscle relaxation, guided imagery, or meditation. Find time to experiment with different activities and pick out those that work best for you, ensuring you have a comfortable seating area, soft lighting, and maybe even some tranquil music or scents.

"I used to feel concerned and wouldn't even get any sleep at times," said Michael, a college student. "Including a daily relaxation routine into my activities has changed it all around." According to him, he starts his day with some deep breathing and visualization. He imagines himself in a serene and quiet environment. Before going to bed, he uses progressive muscle relaxation in the evening. He trains and then relaxes muscle groups to drop all the tension and sleep better.

As Michael continued to put his relaxation first, his anxiety, quality of sleep, and general well-being improved considerably. He was able to be straightforward and productive in his studies, stress resilient, and have a positive spirit even through tough times.

Michael's story represents how relaxation practices hold great promise for supporting mental health and well-being. It is in using the power of the mind with guided imagery and visualization, along with personalized relaxation routines, that we can nurture more peace, resilience, and vitality in the face of life's stressors.

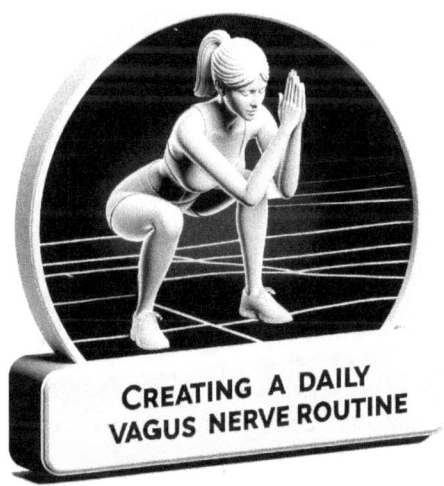

Chapter 15
Creating a Daily Vagus Nerve Exercise Routine

In the complex journey toward optimized health and well-being, consistency is paramount, particularly regarding the vagus nerve, a major component of our autonomic nervous system regulating our stress response, digestive function, heart rate, and overall resilience. Consistency in vagus nerve stimulation techniques has been the key to lasting benefits and improved overall health.

It has been demonstrated that deep breathing, meditation, yoga, and exercise stimulate the vagus nerve and increase the vagal tone, which reduces inflammation, increases the heart rate, and increases stress resilience (Gerritsen & Band, 2018; Breit et al., 2018). In the long run, it's the compounding effect of regular practice: every session builds on the last, creating sustainable changes, not just in the nervous system but also in health in general.

For example, Bhatnagar et al. (2019) concluded that with a regular practice of deep, slow breathing for 5 minutes daily for six weeks, there were significant improvements in heart rate variability and vagal tone in healthy college students. Similarly, Sullivan et al. (2020) indicated that the regular practice of yoga for several weeks or months may massively contribute to improving vagal tone, reduce stress and enhancing well-being.

15.1 Practical Strategies for Maintaining Consistency

It is one thing to understand the need for consistency; it is another thing to practice despite all the demands and distractions of life. To get beyond common obstacles and establish a sound, consistent practice, consider the following strategies:

1. Start small and build incrementally. You may even start with a small commitment of, say, 5 minutes of deep breathing or a short meditation every day. Build up as you gain confidence and the ability to be consistent in your practice.

2. Anchor your practice to existing habits: Take the reins of your vagus nerve practice and anchor it in some habit you already do or routine. For example, you can associate vagus nerve exercises with the morning coffee

or pre-bed wind-down routines. This makes it more automatic and less reliant on willpower or motivation.

3. Design a specific practice space: create a particular space in your home or office for your vagus nerve practice, which will cue your brain that it's time to focus and to work out.

4.List social support: Share your commitment to vagus nerve health as an accountability, encouragement, or motivation strategy to stay consistent with friends, family, or in a supportive group.

Be kind to yourself: Consistency is about showing up and doing the best you can do each day—not about perfection. So, if you miss a practice session, simply acknowledge it without judgment and recommit to your practice the next day.

15.2 Incorporating Breathing Exercises into Your Daily Routine

The power of optimizing vagal nerve health can be in simple, powerful, and accessible tools like breathing exercises. Indeed, many applications have been recently designed that allow conscious control over one's breathing, such as deep belly breathing, breathing through alternate nostrils, and other specifically designed techniques. It turns out that the powerful influence of such techniques on the autonomic nervous system is through the stimulation of the vagus nerve, which reduces stress and anxiety, facilitating a status of calmness and balance.

Certain times of the day are "naturally" good for using breathing practice. This is because they may represent pauses or transitions in our routine where we are likely to be stressed, anxious, or need to be more grounded. Opportune moments for incorporating breathing exercises include:

1. Upon Waking: Start your day off with a few minutes of mindful breathing to establish the day with a feeling of relaxation and clarity.

2. Commuting: Breathe deeply for a few breaths at natural points during your journey, or set aside a specific part to focus on your breath.

3. At your desk: Breathing exercise when you become stressed, overwhelmed, or mentally tired while working or studying.

4. Pre-meal: Take a few deep breaths at the start of each meal to signal your body that it's time to get ready to switch into rest and digest mode.

5. Times of tension or stress: Deep, slow breathing can be utilized to stimulate your parasympathetic nervous system and reduce heart rate and blood pressure, creating a sense of well-being and focus.

6. Before Bedtime: Do a conscious breathing exercise before your bedtime for improved quality of sleep and an increase in relaxation.

Make breathing exercises a sustainable and consistent routine by building up gradually: start small, build on the duration and frequency, link the practice to an existing habit, use cues and visual reminders, hire an accountability partner or get support, and celebrate the small wins on the way.

15.3 Overcoming Obstacles and Maintaining Motivation

Most likely, with the best of intentions and sincere efforts, we all face a little trouble or some impediments in the way of holding a consistent practice of exercises that tone the vagus nerve. Common roadblocks usually include time constraints and competing priorities, lack of immediate results or visibility of progress, boredom or monotony associated with the practice, self-doubt, and negative self-talk.

Below are some ways to overcome these roadblocks and keep yourself motivated:

1. Clarify your "why": Reflect on your deepest aspirations and values. Consider how your practice reflects and supports these overarching goals. Write your "why" statement down, and place it somewhere you'll see it regularly; read it daily as a reminder of the bigger picture of what you're doing.

2. Set Specific and Achievable Goals: Set short- and long-term goals of your vagal practice, making them SMART—specific, measurable, achievable, relevant, time-bound. Celebrate your progress along the way.

3. Create a social environment of support: Contract a family friend to act as a "practice buddy," become involved in an existing community online or geographically, or contract a coach or mentor who will provide instruction, support, and follow-up.

4. Mix it up and keep it fresh: Infuse creativity into the repetitiveness of your vagal exercise routine by trying new techniques or modalities, setting

creative challenges or themes for your practice, and applying a spirit of curiosity and experiment into your daily practice.

5. Be self-compassionate: Develop a strong sense of self-compassion and kindness toward yourself. Remember that setbacks, inconsistencies, and moments of struggle are a common and imperative part of any growth process.

15.4 The Journey Continues

Building a consistent and changing health habit, be it exercises of the vagus nerve or any other practice of self-care or self-discovery, is not a linear or predictable path. There will be moments of ease and flow, as well as moments of challenge and resistance.

Remember that as you walk this trail of health for your Vagus Nerve and transformation of self, challenges and setbacks are not meant to reflect a failure or insufficiency on your part but are instead an invitation to a more profound commitment: a more apparent intention and an opportunity to lean into support and guidance always available to you.

Have faith in your body and mind, in the natural wisdom of nature, in the wisdom of the vagus, all there to bring balance, resilience, and better function of the organism. Bring in the people and practices that make you feel encouraged and inspired, that bring your worthiness and the potential you have to your attention.

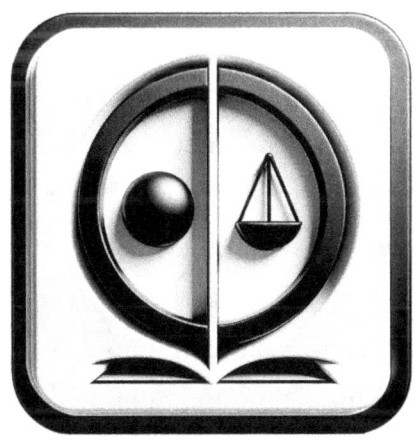

Conclusion

As we approach the end of this journey inside the exciting world of the vagus nerve and its enormous influence on our body, mind, and emotions, I'd like to take a moment to reflect on the central ideas and practices we've passed through and which open themselves to the great potential of change in both our experiences and our lives.

This book is about the autonomic nervous system and how the vagus nerve is critically involved in controlling stress, maintaining an emotional balance, and fostering adaptive responses. We have been reviewing the nuanced but elegant operations of the autonomic nervous system and the integral role of the vagus in regulating stress reactivity, emotional balance, and overall resilience. We have seen the groundbreaking findings of Polyvagal Theory, which shed light on the dynamic interrelations between our physiologic states and our ability to be socially engaged, feel safe, and be connected.

But most important of all, we have learned a goldmine of practical tools and techniques for the stimulation and strengthening of the vagus nerve: a roadmap from simple breathing exercises and mindfulness practices to the power of sound therapy, cold exposure, and physical touch. While offering very different ways of achieving these ends, most modalities attest to creating more profound states of inner peace and vitality, reducing inflammation, and calming the nervous system.

As we have seen, the benefits of vagus nerve activation far exceed physical health. At the same time, this is not a simple story of gargling one's way to emotional resilience, joy, connection, and general well-being and flourishing.

In a world that very often seems like it is too much and very stressful most of the time, the practices and worldviews put forth in this book function as a compass in enabling one to navigate the challenges of life as gracefully and with as much equanimity as possible. They remind us that no matter what the circumstances are, we always have the power to regulate our nervous system, choose our response, and cultivate a more profound sense of safety and wholeness within ourselves.

But the journey with vagal tone is not a one-size-fits-all proposition. Each of us has our own one-of-a-kind history, needs, and goals, and what works for one person will not work for another. That's why it's so important to approach these practices with a spirit of curiosity, experimentation, and self-compassion.

Please play around with the different exercises and techniques we have looked into. Notice how they make you feel and listen deep within yourself, letting your inner guide direct you toward what resonates most with you. Remember: It's not about doing it perfectly; it's about making a gradual and sustainable shift toward balance, resilience, and joy.

As you go toward total well-being, remind yourself that you are not alone. In seeking vagus nerve health, you are in good company with an ever-growing number of individuals who have awakened to the power of transformation through this unique pathway wired physically in their bodies. You are returning to your body, mind, and spirit, which are innately wise and strong.

And as you keep experimenting with and applying these practices to your everyday life, I have complete confidence that you will soon start to feel significantly alive, connected, and on purpose. That is, you will further realize your capability to deal with the ebb and flow of life more quickly and flexibly, to savor the joys and beauty of your life, and to be more fully and authentically present in your relations and life's work.

So let this be an invitation to embrace the power of your vagus nerve, to trust in the incredible capacity for healing and growth that lies within you, and to embark on a lifelong journey to holistic well-being and self-discovery.

Know that wherever you go, you have the ultimate tool for healing, change, and joy: the wisdom held within your incredible vagus nerve.

Last but not least, I'd like to share a few basic yet essential reminders for you to take with you as you journey even further:

- Your nervous system is your superpower: respect it, nurture it, and trust it because it has a remarkable, self-healing recovery capacity.

- There isn't a suitable formula to engage a vagus nerve. Experiment, explore, and find the practices that feel the most joyful, easeful, and alive.

- You are not your thoughts, emotions, or sensations. You are the vast, wide-open awareness that holds them all with love and grace.

- Connect - the key to resilience. Prioritize social support and relationships with others, friends, and yourself.

Healing is not linear; it's just a ride. Embrace it with curiosity, self-compassion, and an open desire to learn about the lows and highs, the struggles and the victories.

Remember, above all, that you are whole, worthy, and immensely resilient—just as you are. Your vagus nerve health is not about fixing or changing who you are; it's about coming home to your most profound, most authentic self and letting that self brighten fully in the world.

So breathe deep, feel the in and out of life within you, and know that within you are all the resources you need to live well right here, right now. Your vagus nerve is your partner, guide, and friend on this spectacular life journey.

I was truly honored to have been part of your journey through this book, and I still do believe that through your trip to the exploration of healing and vagal tone, you will be taken to places that shall be out of the ordinary.

And you will never forget how magnificent, valuable, and powerful you are.

You can place trust in the wisdom and resilience of your beautiful nervous system.

May you come home over and over again to the great love that is within you.

With love, appreciation, and boundless faith in your ability to heal and thrive,

Your friend and fellow traveler on the path of vagus nerve health and holistic well-being.

www.ingramcontent.com/pod-product-compliance
Lightning Source LLC
Chambersburg PA
CBHW052314220526
45472CB00001B/117